Vertigo and dizziness

Lucy Yardley

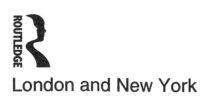

London and New York

First published 1994
by Routledge
11 New Fetter Lane, London EC4P 4EE

Simultaneously published in the USA and Canada
by Routledge
29 West 35th Street, New York, NY 10001

Typeset in Times by LaserScript, Mitcham, Surrey
Printed and bound in Great Britain by
Biddles Ltd, Guildford and King's Lynn

British Library Cataloguing in Publication Data
A catalogue record for this book is available from the British Library

Library of Congress Cataloging in Publication Data
A catalog record for this book has been requested

ISBN 0–415–10209–X

Contents

Editors' preface

Although problems of vertigo and dizziness affect large numbers of people, they are little known about and have not found wide publicity. To experience these difficulties is disturbing and can be alarming. Many individuals so affected not only seek to find treatment, but also search for an explanation of their symptoms.

Dr Yardley has performed pioneering research work in this neglected area. She brings together her own, and others', work in a highly readable book and demonstrates how an appreciation of the psychological and social factors surrounding vertigo and dizziness brings us closer to a comprehensive understanding of their impact on people's lives. Dr Yardley's experience of working clinically with patients and other professionals has contributed to her understanding of the range and complexity of the issues individuals face when they confront these disturbing and disruptive problems, and the effect of advice and treatment.

Dr Yardley's research in this area encompasses both quantitative and qualitative methods of investigation. Together these provide the detailed knowledge necessary to understand patients' perspectives of their problem. The evidence of these methods is apparent in the book, which shows in their own words the difficulties people can experience. Dr Yardley shows a sensitive and perspicacious understanding of vertigo and dizziness, and her book will be of great value to those interested in gaining an understanding of the issues of vertigo and dizziness as they relate to health and psychological and social function. It will be a significant benefit to health care professionals working in the area and also to those with a general interest in problems associated with chronic illness. Just as importantly, it will help to further the understanding of those individuals suffering from problems of vertigo and dizziness who wish to gain an insight into their condition.

Stanton Newman and Ray Fitzpatrick, 1994

Author's preface and acknowledgements

My interest in the problems of people suffering from vertigo (dizziness or imbalance) was awakened by my experience of carrying out diagnostic testing on people with suspected balance system defects. After these patients had waited several months for these tests, and then endured two hours of fairly unpleasant and frightening procedures (during which time they usually confided in me the entire history surrounding their vertigo), they would invariably ask anxiously, 'What is wrong with me? What will happen to me now?' I was as unhappy as they were with the inadequacy of the cautious reply I was often obliged to give: 'The tests have not shown anything seriously wrong with your balance system – the doctor will see you again in another month or two.' The purpose of this book is to provide a more satisfactory and complete answer to their questions, by analysing and explaining the factors which contribute to vertigo and recovery from vertigo.

When I first started to research the topic of dizziness and imbalance I was primarily interested in the perceptual and psychophysiological aspects of disorientation, and I therefore began by exploring individual differences in perceptual, postural and autonomic responses to disorienting conditions. At the same time, I became increasingly aware that the effects on life-style and well-being of which people with vertigo typically complained seemed very far removed from the perceptual-motor difficulties which were supposed to be their 'real' problem, and which constituted the exclusive focus of medical interest and treatment. Interview and questionnaire studies helped me to identify psychosocial, environmental and behavioural elements of the experience of vertigo, and allowed me to begin to construct the more complex, multidimensional description of the experience developed in this book.

I would like to thank numerous friends and colleagues for their support, and in particular Alan Costall, who first inspired me to write this book and guided me through the Ph.D. thesis on which it is based, and whose thoughtful questions and erudite comments have had a profound and enduring influence on my thinking and writing. The series editors, Stan Newman and Ray Fitzpatrick, have also given me invaluable encouragement and sound advice. I am grateful to Linda Luxon and Johanna Beyts for sharing with me their considerable clinical expertise in rehabilitation for people with vertigo. I wish to thank Michelle Lacoudraye-Harter, Alison Todd, Judith Bird, Elaine Masson and Carl Verschuur for their help with collecting and coding the interview and questionnaire material, and also the following people for their interest, advice and practical assistance: Anthony Gale, Roger Ingham, Denise Cafarelli-Dees, Alan Martin, Michael Gresty and Adolfo Bronstein. Finally, I am indebted to everyone who participated in my studies; their graphic and candid accounts are fundamental to the understanding of vertigo which this book hopes to achieve.

1994

Chapter 1

Nature and causes of vertigo

I was standing in my bedroom, brushing my hair in front of the
mirror, and suddenly it was as if I had two heads – me looking at the
mirror and knowing that I was, but the inner head spinning round and
everything going with it.

When you're not near anything you feel as though you don't know
whether you're standing up or laying down or what, because there's
such a vast area around you . . . it was all as though I was standing in
the sea on my own with miles and miles all round me, and there was
nothing to hang on to.

I wake up and everything's black, the room's going round, the bed's
like a boat tossing about, and I'm feeling sick. I usually have to go to
the toilet, be sick, I go all weak and limp, cold. It's the weakness
afterwards too, you feel as though you've been seriously ill, I'm
exhausted, limp, I can't pick up a cup sometimes for a few hours . . .
I get them [attacks] about every five to six weeks, I never know just
when . . . When I have one of my severe turns I don't do anything for
four or five days, I sit like a zombie.

The preceding accounts attempt to convey the confusing, often terrifying, and almost incommunicable experience of people with symptoms
which doctors label 'vertigo'. Sufferers have difficulty finding any
accurate descriptor for their unique phenomenological state, but tend to
use expressions such as 'dizziness', 'whirling', 'a swimming sensation',
'a feeling of unsteadiness or falling'. The medical definition of the term
'vertigo' (which doctors pronounce as 'ver-*tie*-go') is quite different
from the lay usage of this word (ordinarily pronounced '*ver*-tee-go'). In
everyday use, the word vertigo most commonly describes a fear of
heights, although it is sometimes also used to refer to generalised

feelings of giddiness, faintness, confusion, anxiety or insecurity, regardless of the precise nature and cause of these sensations. However, 'vertigo' is strictly defined medically as an illusion of movement of the self or of the environment. This illusion of movement can be caused by any disorder or injury that disrupts the functioning of the multisensory balance system, which controls the perception of orientation and self-motion relative to the external environment. In the medical context, the term 'vertigo' is therefore simply a technical label for the symptom of perceptual disorientation, which can be due to a wide variety of causes.

SCOPE AND PURPOSE OF THIS BOOK

Although vertigo is a common health problem which can cause quite severe disability and distress, there has been surprisingly little research into the impact it has on people's lives. This may be partly due to the perplexity and confusion that surrounds the topic. A firm diagnosis of the organic cause for any particular case of vertigo is frequently difficult to achieve, since there are so many possible aetiologies. Indeed, often it is not possible to even confirm that some physical dysfunction exists, as the functioning of the balance system is extremely complex and difficult to test. The sensations of perceptual disorientation can be vague and difficult to describe, and so symptoms of balance system dysfunction may be mistaken for signs of other physical disorders that can cause dizziness, ranging from hypotension to epilepsy. Alternatively, since dizziness is one of the most common sensations experienced during a panic attack and is included as a symptom in the clinical descriptions of several psychiatric disorders, complaints of dizziness are often interpreted as a sign of underlying anxiety or psychological disturbance. Consequently, there is no neatly defined and circumscribed population of vertigo sufferers available for study, and any attempt to analyse the problem of vertigo is beset by the difficulties pertaining to uncertain diagnoses and diverse aetiologies.

Owing to these diagnostic problems, the population of people who complain of vertigo undoubtedly encompasses a variety of individuals, ranging from those with severe disorders of the balance system to those with no clinically significant physical abnormalities. It is possible that the experience of vertigo is similar, whether the origin of the feelings of disorientation is primarily physical or psychological. The fears, uncertainties, social embarrassment, occupational problems, and the form and extent of the malaise and handicap resulting from spells of dizziness caused by anxiety may be comparable in many respects to the difficulties encountered by people suffering from organic disorders. Indeed, recent studies have shown not only that the symptoms and problems of many people subject to panic attacks are very similar to those of people with balance system disorders (Jacob *et al.* forthcoming), but also that subtle abnormalities of perceptual-motor function are common among people with panic and agoraphobia (Yardley *et al.* 1994b). None the less, the scope of this book is deliberately limited to consideration of the experience of individuals who are believed to have some organic balance system dysfunction. In the studies upon which much of this book is based, this criterion was met by including only those individuals who had received a firm diagnosis of peripheral vestibular disorder from an experienced hospital clinician. In addition, the homogeneity of the samples obtained in this way was assured by comparing the characteristics of the people who exhibited definite signs of balance system dysfunction upon examination and testing (usually slightly more than half of the sample) with those who did not. Since absolutely no differences in diagnosis, symptoms, handicap or psychosocial profile were found between people who did or did not show objective signs of organic dysfunction, it seems reasonable to conclude that the failure to obtain evidence of balance system dysfunction in the remaining cases was simply due to the limitations of the available tests (discussed in the following chapter).

There are two principal reasons why I have chosen to focus selectively upon the experience of disorientation known to be caused by physical disorder, despite the possibility that there may be important parallels with the experience of people whose dizziness is due primarily to psychological factors. The first is that feelings of disorientation are all too readily categorised as 'all in the mind' by professionals working within both medicine and psychology. The psychological explanations for symptoms of vague dizziness are so well established that the sometimes subtle and complex perceptual causes for disorientation may be overlooked. Moreover, there is a prevalent (albeit unproven) hypothesis, familiar to all clinicians who treat vertiginous patients, that some forms of vertigo due to organic dysfunction may have a partly psychosomatic aetiology and that vertigo sufferers are therefore likely to have neurotic personalities, or a predisposition for anxiety and hypochondria. Consequently, the reported psychosocial problems of even those people who obtain a diagnosis of physical disorder may be regarded as signs of emotional distress or personality disorder. One of the purposes of this book is to present an alternative to these interpretations of the link between anxiety and vertigo, by describing precisely how and why people who were previously psychologically healthy and emotionally stable may become seriously distressed and handicapped because of recurrent attacks of vertigo due to disordered balance system functioning.

The second reason for basing this book entirely on studies of people with a diagnosis of balance system dysfunction is to illustrate the way in which the activities, attitudes, intentions and environment of the individual fundamentally affect the experience of vertigo, even when it *is* clearly due to some organic disorder. The importance of cognitive and behavioural responses to events and environments is readily accepted in the context of 'non-organic' complaints of disorientation, such as the dizziness and confusion which are often experienced during a panic attack. However, the essential role of such processes is seldom fully appreciated in the case of individuals diagnosed as suffering from vertigo caused by organic disorder; in the attempt to identify and remediate the pathophysiological features of these patients' problems, other equally important and intrinsic features of their experience of illness are often ignored. Hence, although evidence of an organic disorder was requisite for inclusion in the studies of dizziness on which this book is based, the organic dysfunction is not regarded as being necessarily either the primary or the central feature of the experience of disorientation.

The following chapters detail the way in which physiological processes mutually affect and are affected by attitudes, activities and environments, and demonstrate how the experience and course of vertigo emerges from combined and reciprocal influences, both physical and psychosocial, and both internal and external to the individual concerned. Chapter 2 examines the psychosocial consequences of the diagnostic and prognostic uncertainty which typically surrounds vertigo. In Chapter 3 the practical and psychological repercussions of the physical disability associated with vertigo and dizziness are considered. Analysis of the processes determining the nature and extent of disability shows how both environmental factors and the activities and perceptual-motor skills of the individual can contribute to disorientation and to the recovery of equilibrium. The fourth chapter explores the association between anxiety and dizziness, and describes a variety of psychophysiological, cognitive-behavioural and neuropsychological mechanisms which might mediate a bi-directional causal relationship between the emotional and perceptual aspects of disorientation. Chapter 5 portrays the social impact of vertigo, and examines the way in which the reactions of friends and strangers, employers and colleagues, partners and children may aggravate or ameliorate the handicap and distress caused by vertigo. Finally, the process of adaptation, adjustment and recovery is analysed and the potential benefits of various types of therapy considered.

In order to appreciate how environmental, cognitive, emotional and behavioural factors can affect the course of vertigo, a basic under-standing of the neurophysiology and biomechanics of the balance system is first required. The remainder of this chapter therefore provides an elementary description of the balance system, and of the charac-teristics and common organic causes of vertigo. (For more detailed descriptions of the pathophysiology and differential diagnosis of vertigo, the reader is referred to Brandt 1991; Dix and Hood 1984; Wright 1988.)

THE BALANCE SYSTEM

The perception and control of orientation and self-motion is achieved by integrating information from three primary sources: the *visual, somato-sensory* (or proprioceptive) and *vestibular* sensory systems. The *visual* system can derive constant feedback about self-motion from the movement of the environment across the visual field. For example, turning the head to the left produces a simultaneous equal and opposite movement of the entire visual scene to the right. Similarly, when falling forwards the sight of the ground rushing up to meet the eyes precedes any bodily sensation induced by impact with the ground. The *somatosensory* system comprises all the sensors in the body; sensors in the muscles and joints provide information about the position of the head, trunk and limbs and internally controlled movements, while sensors in the skin register direct contact with the environment. For instance, when an individual turns to the left the somato-sensory system monitors the joint and muscle activity involved in making the turn, while information about contact with the ground is obtained from the soles of the feet. Finally, the *vestibular* system directly senses the acceleration and orientation of the head. Although the vestibular system is not the most important source of information relating to self-motion – in most situations, the visual and somatosensory systems actually provide more precise and reliable information – disorders of the vestibular system are the most common organic cause of illusions of movement. The functioning of the vestibular system will therefore be described in more detail below.

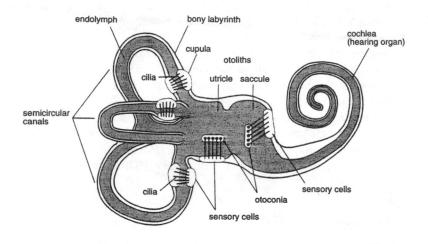

Figure 1 Schematic diagram of the key elements of the vestibular organ

The vestibular system

The peripheral vestibular sensory organ forms part of the inner ear, and consists of a tiny bony structure (the 'labyrinth') filled with two types of fluid, known as perilymph and endolymph (see Figure 1). The vestibular organ comprises the *semicircular canals*, which detect angular acceleration, and the *otoliths*, which monitor linear acceleration and the orientation of the head relative to gravity.

The *otoliths* contain 'cilia', which are similar to stiff hairs and stick out of the sensory cells of the otolith. When the cilia are in their resting position, the sensory cells give out a constant signal, or 'resting discharge' of neural activity. However, when the cilia are bent this signal changes, as the neural activity either increases or decreases, depending upon the direction in which the cilia are deflected. At the opposite end from the sensory cells, the cilia are attached to a membrane in which are embedded minute but relatively heavy crystals ('otoconia'). When the orientation of the head changes (see Figure 2), the sensory cells move with the head, to which they are firmly attached, but the heavy, free-floating membrane containing the otoconia lags behind. Consequently, the cilia are bent, and a change in the sensory

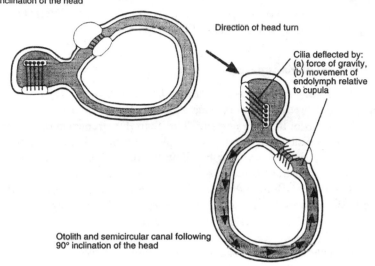

Otolith and semicircular canal before 90° inclination of the head

Direction of head turn

Cilia deflected by:
(a) force of gravity,
(b) movement of endolymph relative to cupula

Otolith and semicircular canal following 90° inclination of the head

Figure 2 Schematic representation of the biomechanical effects of a ninety degree (forward) inclination of the head

signal is produced. These alterations in the sensory signal can be produced either by a change in the position of the head relative to the force of gravity, or by the force of linear acceleration or deceleration, such as that produced by stopping in a car (horizontal force) or in a lift (vertical force). The otoliths consist of two structures – the utricle and saccule – which are set approximately at right angles, so that both vertical and horizontal forces can be detected.

The *semicircular canals* are three ring-like bony tubes protruding from the utricle. A small swelling ('ampulla') at one end of each semicircular canal contains sensory cells and cilia similar to those in the otoliths, but in this case the cilia extend towards the 'cupula', a piece of tissue which virtually fills the ampulla. When the head accelerates in the same (angular) direction as the plane of the semicircular canal (see Figure 2), all the structures of the semicircular canal naturally move with the head. However, owing to inertia the fluid (endolymph) which fills the canal lags behind the head movement, and therefore flows against the cilia, bending them and thereby producing a change in the signal emitted by the sensory cells. The three semicircular canals are positioned at right angles, so that between them they can detect acceleration in each of the three possible planes of motion, both lateral (spinning) and vertical (somersaults and cartwheels).

Central vestibular interconnections

Signals relating to linear and angular accelerations detected by the two otoliths and three semicircular canals pass via the vestibular nerve to the vestibular nuclei in the brain-stem. The central interconnections within the balance system are extremely complex; information from the vestibular organs in both ears is combined with information derived (mainly) from vision and the somatosensory system at various levels within the brain-stem, cerebellum and cortex. This integrated information provides the basis not only for the conscious perception of orientation and self-motion, but also the pre-conscious control of eye movements and posture, by means of what are known as the vestibulo-ocular and vestibulo-spinal reflexes. The purpose of the vestibulo-ocular reflex is to maintain a stable point of visual fixation during head movement by automatically compensating for the head movement with an equivalent eye movement in the opposite direction. Without an efficient vestibulo-ocular reflex the world would appear to jump about during rapid head movements; people with poor vestibulo-ocular reflexes often complain that their environment seems to bob up and down when they walk along. The vestibulo-spinal reflexes help to control posture and maintain an upright orientation.

BALANCE SYSTEM DYSFUNCTION AND VERTIGO

In normal circumstances, the perceptual information about orientation derived from the vestibular, visual and somatosensory systems is congruent. In other words, when we turn our head the visual field sweeps past our eyes, the vestibular system signals angular acceleration, and at the same time information from our neck muscles and joints confirms that our head is actively turning. Indeed, when the balance system is functioning properly there is no conscious awareness of 'sensations' corresponding to the perception of orientation – we just automatically register our precise orientation and self-motion and utilise this information to maintain balance and well-coordinated activity. However, when an apparent mismatch occurs between the different sensory inputs to the balance system, the perceptual uncertainty this creates is itself experienced as a sensation, which may be described as dizziness, disorientation, or vertigo. The perceptual disorientation can be caused either by a failure of sensory processing, or by man-made environmental conditions which our balance system has not been equipped by evolution to cope with, such as passive transport by car, boat, aeroplane, or even spaceship (the space sickness caused by floating around in conditions of weightlessness causes significant problems for astronauts, particularly when wearing their helmets!). If the disorientation is attributable to internal dysfunction it is labelled 'vertigo', whereas disorientation caused by external perceptual conditions is known as 'motion sickness' (or more specifically, car-sickness, sea-sickness, etc.).

The pathophysiological causes of vertigo include dysfunction of any of the sensory systems contributing to orientation perception, or of the central interconnections of the balance system; these disorders and their effects are described in more detail in the following section. The environmental causes comprise any situation characterised by an unusual combination of visual, vestibular and somatosensory information. For example, when a person in a ship travelling across rough seas sits in a cabin with no portholes, the vestibular system will signal constant motion, but this information is contradicted by the inability of the visual system to detect any corresponding movement of the visual field since the visual environment (the cabin) moves with the ship and passenger. These relatively uncommon perceptual conditions are experienced as disorientation and sea-sickness, since on dry land vestibular signals are usually accompanied by visual field motion. (Of course, there are many other types and combinations of perceptual information that can result in motion sickness at sea, on land and in the air; for a more detailed discussion of the factors contributing to motion sickness see Crampton 1990; Yardley 1992.)

Many of the symptoms of vertigo are very similar to those of motion sickness, as one might expect in view of their shared causal origin. The defining symptom is, as previously stated, an illusion of movement. However, the subjective experience of people who receive a diagnosis of 'vertigo' can be extremely varied, as the following descriptions illustrate:

The floors start to come up and things revolve and you feel nausea . . . you just entirely lose your balance and sort of reel about.

Every time I looked down all I could see was a black hole in front of me – everything seems to come pushing me back.

> I was beginning to sweat, would feel cold, shivery, I would physically begin to look pale, drained.

> I go on the tilt, it washes over my head, surges through – a bit like if you went up one of these loop things, Alton Towers [a roller-coaster ride] or something like that.

The classic symptom of acute vestibular imbalance is a strong sensation of spinning, or of the environment whirling around. However, there may be simply a momentary feeling of being pushed to one side, an impression that the world appears to be rocking or moving about, or just a vague consciousness of giddiness or unsteadiness. The perceptual disorientation also results in two constellations of secondary symptoms. The first group of symptoms are directly attributable to the disruption of ocular and postural control caused by balance system dysfunction. Disordered vestibulo-ocular reflexes can result in a blurred or flickering visual image and difficulty in focusing, while abnormal vestibulo-spinal reflexes may cause staggering, loss of balance and falling, or a tendency to veer to one side when walking. In addition, disorientation triggers a range of autonomic changes. The principal symptoms are nausea, vomiting, pallor and cold sweating, but other common physiological concomitants of vertigo and motion sickness include salivation, flatulence or diarrhoea, sighing or yawning, a feeling of warmth, an increase in heart rate and respiration rate, headache, drowsiness and fatigue, apathy, anxiety and depression. Many of these secondary physiological changes are undoubtedly triggered directly via central pathways (Jacob *et al.* 1992), although anxiety may contribute to or exacerbate some of this autonomic symptomatology (see Chapter 4).

While perceptual disorientation and failure of vestibulo-ocular and postural co-ordination are simply the inevitable consequence of a disruption of balance system functioning, the adaptive significance or 'survival value' of the ancillary autonomic symptoms remains the subject of speculation. Triesman (1977) has proposed an 'evolutionary hypothesis' to account for motion sickness which may also be considered relevant to the autonomic symptomatology provoked by vertigo. He suggested that motion sickness is simply an accidental manifestation of what originally evolved as an adaptive response to ingesting poisons which disrupt co-ordination and perception through their effects on the central nervous system. The vomiting would expel the poison, and the nausea would cause aversion to the poisonous substance; indeed, sensitivity and aversion to sights and smells associated with periods of disorientation has been observed in both motion sickness (Lawther and

Griffin 1988) and vertigo (Grisby and Johnston 1989). The general lethargy and malaise associated with both motion sickness and vertigo would tend to limit the amount of activity undertaken while the animal was dangerously uncoordinated.

However severe the symptoms initially provoked by peripheral sensory dysfunction, neurophysiological and sensorimotor adaptation to this dysfunction can gradually be achieved by means of a process of 'habituation' or 'compensation', provided that the central structures and interconnections within the balance system are functioning normally. At first, the change in the sensory signal resulting from, say, the sudden complete destruction of the vestibular organ in the left ear will result in a strong sensation of spinning to the left, because the resting discharge from the right vestibular organ is no longer counterbalanced by signals from the left vestibular organ. Similarly, there will be a tendency to veer or fall towards the left side, and the eyes will tend to drift over to the left. As an 'emergency' measure, central processes automatically attempt partially to suppress the remaining vestibular input. In the longer term, compensation is achieved by a process of perceptual relearning; the balance system adjusts to the fact that there is now no vestibular input from the left side, and utilises information from the healthy vestibular organ and from vision and the somatosensory system to substitute for the missing vestibular signal. This process of relearning can only occur through repeated experience of the new pattern of sensory information that is now provoked by each head movement and orientation.

The subjective experience of this process of compensation is that the person who suffers unilateral vestibular failure will immediately learn to lie down and keep absolutely still, in order to minimise the changes in vestibular activity which provoke dizziness and nausea. After several hours, the disorientation when lying still will lessen, but the slightest head movement will provoke fresh symptoms. Over time the person will be forced to make some repeated head movements (e.g. lifting or turning the head), and eventually the disorientation provoked by these movements will become less severe, as the balance system learns the new pattern of information associated with these movements. However, new movements, such as bending down or nodding quickly, will continue to provoke dizziness until they have been repeated enough times for the process of adjustment to occur. In this sense, the process of adaptation to sensory dysfunction is very similar to the acquisition of 'sea-legs'. During a short sea passage there is insufficient time for the balance system to adjust to the new pattern of perceptual information experienced on a ship, and the individual will tend to stagger as the ship heaves, and may feel very ill. However, over the course of a longer voyage the continued exposure to these perceptual conditions eventually results in complete adaptation, and the same individual is able to move around freely and without sickness.

INCIDENCE AND COMMON ORGANIC CAUSES OF VERTIGO

The precise incidence of vertigo due to balance system dysfunction is very difficult to ascertain because of the problems associated with defining and diagnosing the condition. The exact prevalence of cases of vertigo within the community, and the proportion of these that are actually seen in general practice or referred to hospital, is therefore unknown. It is also difficult to establish the relative prevalence of the various causes of vertigo; although some clinicians have detailed the incidence of various disorders within their specific clinic populations (e.g. Drachman and Hart 1972), these figures are likely to be heavily influenced by local customs relating to referral and diagnosis. Nevertheless, it is known that each year five out of every thousand people in the UK population seek consultations with their doctor because of symptoms which are classified by their general practitioner as true vertigo, and a further ten people are seen by their general practitioner on account of a complaint of dizziness or giddiness (RCGP/OPCS 1986). A recent survey in North America (Kroenke 1992) found that one in four people reported that they had experienced dizziness at some time, and in 80 per cent of these cases the dizziness had been sufficiently severe to result in handicap and/or motivate recourse to medical assistance. Although vertigo can affect people of any age, the incidence rises with advancing age owing to the greater prevalence in older people of disorders which can give rise to vertigo (such as cardiovascular and cerebrovascular disease). In a community survey of people aged 50–65, a quarter of the sample stated that they *currently* suffered from giddiness or dizziness (Stephens 1990), while by the age of 80 years two-thirds of women and one-third of men report having experienced episodes of vertigo (Luxon 1984). Baloh (1992) notes that dizziness is the most common presenting complaint in primary care among people aged over 74.

The symptoms and prognosis in cases of vertigo vary according to the aetiology. A brief overview of the major causes of vertigo, together with typical symptoms and prognoses, is therefore given below. However, the distinctions between these disorders are not always entirely clear-cut and there can be a considerable overlap in symptomatology.

For example, episodic vertigo may be associated with a feeling of fullness in the ears but no hearing loss or tinnitus, Ménière's disease is sometimes preceded by accident or infection and accompanied by signs of benign paroxysmal positional vertigo, while a vague dizziness may persist in the intervals between attacks of definite positional vertigo.

Peripheral vestibular causes of vertigo

One of the most common types of vertigo is known variously as 'vestibular neuronitis', 'labyrinthitis', or sometimes 'epidemic' or 'idiopathic' vertigo, and is characterised by the classic symptoms of vestibular dysfunction described in the previous section, often preceded by a viral infection. The exact definition of the disorder and its precise cause, or causes, are not fully established, but the recorded incidence in one general practice was 1.7 cases per thousand people per year (Cooper 1993). Another very common vestibular disorder is known as 'benign paroxysmal positional vertigo'. This is thought to occur when heavy debris (otoconia), dislodged from the otoliths as a result of age-related degeneration or head injury, comes to rest in one of the semicircular canals. The affected canal therefore starts to register changes in orientation relative to gravity, but continues to signal angular acceleration. The subjective experience is that changes in orientation, such as lying down or rolling over in bed, can provoke a brief but extremely powerful sensation of spinning (and accompanying nausea). Both vestibular neuronitis and benign positional paroxysmal vertigo usually clear up spontaneously over a period of weeks or months, but an unfortunate minority of individuals find that they have repeated attacks or persistent symptoms for many years.

The major cause of recurrent attacks of severe vertigo is a syndrome known as 'Ménière's disease', which is characterised by a unique combination of symptoms: severe bouts of vertigo lasting several hours; fluctuating tinnitus (a noise in the ear or head) – generally a low-pitched buzzing or roaring in one ear, which at first accompanies attacks of vertigo but may later become continuous; an intermittent feeling of pressure in the ear; fluctuating, progressive unilateral hearing impairment, which interferes predominantly with hearing for low-pitched sounds initially, but may eventually result in complete loss of hearing in the affected ear. These symptoms are generally thought to arise as a result of an imbalance of fluid pressures in the inner ear known as 'endolymphatic hydrops', but although evidence of a link between Ménière's disease and hydrops has been found at post-mortem (Rauch *et al.* 1989) the association is not clear-cut since many people with signs of hydrops are asymptomatic. The prognosis for people with Ménière's disease is uncertain, although Browning (1991) calculates that in the long term (over more than a decade) 98 per cent of those seen in hospital clinics recover from their vertigo. Some people have only a few attacks, followed by complete remission. Often acute attacks occur several times a year, and unless complete compensation for the change in the vestibular signal caused by these acute attacks is achieved, the individual may experience considerable residual dizziness and movement-provoked vertigo in the intervening months. The disorder eventually seems to 'burn itself out', usually leaving the sufferer with a permanent unilateral hearing loss and tinnitus but no vertigo, but sometimes the disease spreads later to the previously unaffected ear. Ménière's disease is most common among people aged between 30 and 50 years, with a slight predominance of females, and prevalence estimates range from 0.1 to 1 per cent of the population.

Miscellaneous additional causes of vertigo of peripheral vestibular origin include a variety of disorders and diseases of the middle ear, ototoxic drugs (used only in medical emergencies), obstruction of the peripheral blood vessels supplying the inner ear, syphilis, herpes zoster, or fracture of the temporal bone. Occasionally, a small hole ('fistula') in the membrane of the vestibular organ can be caused by middle ear disease, surgery, head injury, or the abrupt pressure changes which may be induced by diving, flying, or strenuous physical activity. The hole will allow the fluid inside the organ to leak out ('perilymph leak'), resulting in symptoms of sudden vertigo and unilateral hearing loss, often exacerbated by additional pressure changes (e.g. sneezing) which force the fluid out of the inner ear. Very rarely, vertigo may be due to a benign tumour ('acoustic neuroma') which can develop on the audiovestibular nerve, affecting not only the nerve function but also the blood supply to the inner ear, and eventually pressing upon the brain-stem.

Non-vestibular peripheral causes of vertigo

Disorders of the neck, which may alter the somatosensory information relating to head movement or interfere with the blood supply to the vestibular system, are believed by many clinicians to be a cause of vertigo; common aetiologies include whip-lash injury and cervical spondylosis. Sometimes unsteadiness is related to a loss of feeling in the feet and legs due to 'neuropathy', which may be caused by diabetes, alcohol abuse, vitamin deficiency, damage to the spinal cord, or a number of other disorders. Occasionally the origin of feelings of giddiness, unsteadiness or illusory movement of the environment can be traced to some distortion of the visual input. An abnormal visual input may be caused by weakness of the eye muscles, or may be experienced when adjusting to powerful lenses (such as those worn after an operation to remove cataracts) or to bifocal glasses.

Central causes of vertigo

Although most cases of vertigo are attributable to peripheral (mainly vestibular) pathology, symptoms of disorientation can be caused by a wide range of central disorders or injuries, at the level of the brain-stem, cerebellum or cortex. Vertigo of central origin is almost always accompanied by some other symptom of central neurological disorder, such as sensations of pain, tingling or numbness in the face or limbs, difficulty speaking or swallowing, headache, visual disturbances, and loss of motor control or loss of consciousness. The more common central causes of vertigo include disorders of the blood supply to the brain (ranging from migraine to strokes), epilepsy, multiple sclerosis, alcoholism, and sometimes tumours. Dizziness and imbalance have also been reported as a potential temporary side-effect of a vast array of drugs, including widely used analgesics, contraceptives, and drugs used in the control of cardiovascular disease, diabetes and Parkinson's disease, and in particular the centrally acting drugs such as stimulants, sedatives, anti-convulsants, anti-depressants and tranquillisers (Ballantyne and Ajodhia 1984).

Age-related causes of vertigo

The incidence of vertigo, as noted previously, is age related; there is a progressive growth in the number of reported and diagnosed cases with increasing age. As in the case of age-related hearing loss, it is possible that vertigo in the elderly may be partly attributable to non-specific degeneration within the peripheral and/or central levels of the vestibular system. In addition, many of the disorders which can give rise to vertigo, such as cerebrovascular disease or cervical damage, are more common in the elderly. Often people in the older age-groups are obliged to take a number of medications which can cause dizziness. Finally, disorientation and unsteadiness may result from what is known as 'multisensory dysfunction', a combination of minor defects in the various sensory systems contributing to orientation. For example, failing eyesight alone may not be sufficient to cause imbalance, but the addition of slightly reduced sensation in the lower limbs and intermittent positional vertigo may result in a dangerous and severely handicapping degree of postural instability. Since compensation for vestibular dysfunction requires intact central neurological functioning, alternative sources of sensory input (to substitute for absent or distorted vestibular signals), and plenty of active sensorimotor experience, the process of compensation may sometimes be retarded in the elderly as a result of minor central dysfunction, multisensory impairment, or inadequate physical activity.

Chapter 2

Vertigo and the medical profession

This chapter traces the 'medical careers' of people with vertigo – in other words, the histories of their contact with the medical system and its influence on their experience of illness. The first two sections examine the considerations that initially motivate the decision to seek medical help, and the factors that influence doctors' reactions to complaints of dizziness or vertigo. The third and fourth sections describe experiences of clinical testing, diagnosis and medical treatment. A recurring theme throughout the chapter is the uncertainty which bedevils attempts to explain, predict or treat symptoms of disorientation, and which colours the attitudes of both doctors and patients.

INITIAL EXPERIENCES OF VERTIGO AND THE DECISION TO SEEK MEDICAL HELP

For some people, the onset of a vertigo attack is sudden and violent:

> I thought, 'Oh, I'm feeling a bit dizzy, I must be hungry or some such' . . . within half an hour I couldn't stand.

> I walked into a house and I felt perfectly all right, and suddenly I thought, 'I'm going to be sick.' By the time I got to the loo I couldn't stand up straight. I was literally trembling, I shook all over. I went hot and cold, I burst into tears . . . I just sort of went and fell over.

> I thought I was dying, everything was spinning, spinning round, I was so violently sick. I went back to bed and it carried on for twenty-four hours.

When the attacks of vertigo are as severe and unexpected as in these descriptions, family, friends, or colleagues are usually sufficiently concerned to seek medical assistance at once on behalf of the afflicted individual. When attacks occur at work or in a public place a medical professional or even an ambulance may be summoned, while at home the spouse will generally call in the local doctor. Even if the attacks are not witnessed, the response of most sufferers themselves to such a frightening and bewildering experience is to turn to the medical profession for an immediate definition and explanation of what is happening, as well as prevention, or at least control, of the unpleasant sensations and incapacitation. Consequently, those individuals who initially have acute attacks may pass very quickly through the processes necessary to arrive at a diagnosis of their condition, as in the following account:

> I was in a hotel and I got up in the middle of the night, fell on the floor, and the whole world started to spin. I phoned my wife who got the doctor out. He thought I was drunk or something, but he took the blood pressure and everything and they were normal, so he had a second little thought about it and said to me you might have Ménière's . . . In the next three weeks I had some terrible attacks, in fact I was so bad one night the doctor put me in hospital and then I went through the tests, you know the usual things – I am assuming they eliminate everything, if you haven't got a brain tumour or heart disease they blame it on to Ménière's, and that is exactly what they did.

However, for many people the initial experiences of vertigo are less striking and distinctive. Consequently, there may be a long period during which the symptoms are monitored and their significance assessed without any recourse to medical opinion. Some of the factors and processes which may affect individuals' interpretations of their own symptoms are outlined in Leventhal's 'self-regulatory' model of illness cognition (Leventhal et al. 1980). Leventhal suggests that when confronted by abnormal physical sensations people seek to define their condition using a label, which can be either an illness or an emotion. When the symptoms are unfamiliar, contextual cues may have a particularly strong influence on symptom interpretation; for example, the presence of recent or imminent sources of stress may lead people to attribute their symptoms to anxiety (Baumann et al. 1989).

The accounts given by many of my interviewees of their initial reactions to vertigo certainly indicate that the experience is interpreted in the light of situational factors. Sometimes the disorientation itself may not be perceived as the most prominent or central symptom, so that sufferers develop explanations for malaise which are based primarily on the ancillary symptoms rather than the vertigo itself, and see the vertigo as a secondary symptom of some more familiar ailment:

I developed a terrible headache, I just couldn't sit in the car, my head wanted to fall to the side and I was getting giddy . . . I just at the time assumed it was a very bad headache or in fact a migraine.

I thought I'd had too much sun because I'd been laid out in the sun all day, and that started off everything just moving about, and I was sick and I had this headache, and I thought, 'Oh, I've had too much sun.'

The first time I got it, I was driving long-distance. I thought it was because I was concentrating, using the brain so much on the motorway . . . I started getting the head going round and round and I vomited. I thought it was an upset stomach or something.

Alternatively, when the initial sensations of vertigo are vague and mild they are often dismissed as the effects of stress or fatigue:

The first time I was in the kitchen preparing the evening meal. I move very quickly most of the time and I turned round and I felt dizzy – not exactly dizziness, but veering to one side as if I was going to the right all the time. I just thought I was tired, my mind was on other things, and I should pull myself together and concentrate.

I remember the first one very clearly . . . We went to the school for him [the son] to show me around and we got to the top floor, and quite suddenly I was attacked by giddiness and I couldn't stand up at all. It wasn't a question of height, that had nothing to do with it, and I wasn't looking down a well or anything. My husband and son between them had to get me down and I was very, very sick . . . at the time I didn't connect it at all with the trauma of [the son] going away, it's only afterwards with people having said to me that's what it was that makes me connect them even. I simply thought, we'd had a bit of a day and I was worked up, and I was frightened of making him ashamed of me by being sick upstairs.

This last account conveys particularly clearly the problem posed for vertigo sufferers by the ambiguity of their symptoms, and by their connotations, which include height phobia and emotional distress. In the case of vertigo, the problems associated with deciding whether the condition should be defined as an illness are exacerbated by the vague and intermittent nature of symptoms, and the absence of any well-known label for the experience, such as flu or indigestion. Moreover, apart from vomiting, there are generally none of the customary visible signs of disease, such as a rash, fever, catarrh, or coughing.

The uncertain status of symptoms such as vertigo and dizziness not only causes subjective uncertainty and disquiet, but may also lead to social difficulties:

> The main thing is that as it's not a visible thing therefore you know someone is sorry and all that, but you can tell that they just don't understand how you're feeling. You can't go somewhere, or you can't do this, can't do that – people tend to think that you just don't *want* to go.

> In the early stages she [a colleague at work] thought I was pulling a fast one . . . they used to think it was funny [i.e. suspicious] at work because I was fine that day, and I'd go back the next day perfectly well, but I'd had perhaps just the one day off.

In his analysis of the way in which people evaluate signs of illness, Locker (1981) notes that it is socially requisite that claims of illness are legitimated either by observable manifestations or by accepted (i.e. medical) authority; only then will failure to fulfil normal roles and responsibilities be sanctioned. Consequently, one of the motivations for seeking medical advice may be to try to resolve the uncertainty concerning whether these symptoms represent true 'illness', and to combat suspicions of weakness or malingering by obtaining verification of the existence of a physical disorder. Indeed, formal certification of illness may be essential if the vertigo is interfering with occupational duties, for example by necessitating absence from work or avoidance of heights.

If the vertigo causes no significant social difficulties with family or friends and does not create problems at work, then the individual may not perceive any advantage in consulting a doctor. From the incidence figures given in the preceding chapter, it is evident that only a relatively small minority of cases of vertigo are ever brought to the doctor; whereas between a quarter and a half of middle-aged and elderly people report episodes of giddiness, fewer than one in a hundred people see their local doctor each year with a complaint of vertigo. This does not, of course, mean that vertigo causes no problems at all for those who do not seek medical assistance. Although there have been, perhaps surprisingly, no detailed community studies of the distress or disability resulting from untreated vertigo, the long histories of difficulties described by many people who do eventually seek medical help suggest that at least some of those who are reluctant to complain to their doctor experience a degree of anxiety or handicap on account of vertigo. Indeed, Kroenke (1992) argues that unreported, chronic dizziness is the most likely explanation for the discrepancy between the annual incidence of new cases of dizziness recorded by doctors in the USA (1.8 per cent) and the prevalence of dizziness in the community assessed by self-report (17 per cent). It is likely that, as in the case of hearing loss (Herbst and Humphrey 1981), an attitude of resignation is commonly adopted, and the vertigo is simply tolerated as a minor annoyance or viewed as an unavoidable consequence of ageing. This stoic acceptance of disability may nevertheless have detrimental effects in so far as it prevents the individual from gaining access to potentially beneficial treatment or rehabilitation (Gray 1983). In addition, prolonged minor levels of disability may have unfortunate secondary consequences; for example, giddiness in the elderly may eventually contribute to loss of mobility and dangerous falls (Overstall 1983).

In many cases, medical advice is only sought when the symptoms persist or worsen, but sometimes complaints of quite severe vertigo only come to light when the sufferer visits the doctor on account of a quite different symptom, although this may later prove to be related to the vertigo (for example, headache, hearing loss or tinnitus). Alternatively, consultation may be motivated by some change in circumstances; one person interviewed in the course of my research saw his doctor because he wanted to learn to drive and was worried that vertigo might render him unfit, while another sought medical reassurance that the condition was not a sign of some serious hereditary disease, as she wished to start a family. Nevertheless, in both these cases it is clear that in addition to the immediate and explicit incentive to seek a medical opinion, there must have been some degree of underlying concern about the nature and significance of the disorder. Anxiety about the cause of the vertigo, and the possibility that it is a symptom of some serious illness, is very often the primary motivation for consulting the doctor:

> The fear that it's there and what is it? That is the bottom line – what's wrong?

> I just didn't know what was happening to me. I think you think of the worst thing – I thought that there was something serious wrong and any minute I was going to pop off.

In contrast, in the case of the woman cited below, anxiety about the sinister implications of symptoms of vertigo actually deterred her from consulting a doctor at first, although the combined impact on her life-style of both anxiety and disability eventually prompted her to seek help:

I initially thought, 'What is going on in my head?' You worry about tumours and goodness knows what else, and, you know, it is frightening. You tend to think the worst and I think initially I didn't really go outside too much for information . . . it has just gone on and on, and I think I must have started avoiding things. Worrying about it till eventually I thought, 'I can't take this any more, it is affecting my life too much, it is interfering with my life too much, every aspect of my life.'

In summary, those people who do consult their doctor on account of vertigo appear to do so in order, first, to obtain confirmation of illness and a label for their condition, second, for explanation and reassurance concerning the nature, cause and implications of their symptoms, and finally, in order to obtain relief from their discomfort and alleviation of their disability. Unfortunately, as the following sections will relate, many people who turn to the medical profession for help encounter a variety of obstacles which impede the fulfilment of these aspirations.

DOCTORS' REACTIONS TO DIZZINESS

Doctors' attitudes to vertigo and its management are, of course, as varied as the responses of sufferers themselves, and are heavily influenced by the characteristics of the complaint and of the patient. Nevertheless, in order to arrive at a broadly representative impression of the mainstream medical approach to vertigo in the UK, my own personal observation of the management of vertigo (obtained through several years' experience of clinical audio-vestibulology) was supplemented by systematic sampling of three different sources of information. The first comprised all of the recent (post-1980) textbooks kept in the library of a university teaching hospital, which included sections on vertigo. The second consisted of descriptions of the experiences of medical management derived from a series of interviews with patients from several different hospital clinics, while the third source was responses to a questionnaire survey of 100 consecutive patients seen at a specialist regional centre.

Review of the medical textbooks on vertigo gives an overwhelming impression that the priority is to achieve differential diagnosis of the precise pathology responsible for the complaints of dizziness. Of course, accurate diagnosis is always a medical priority, since the diagnosis generally contains essential information about the nature and likely prognosis of the disorder, and provides the rationale for the selection of a particular course of treatment. Nevertheless, it is remarkable that in the case of vertigo the textbooks are almost entirely devoted to descriptions of the symptoms and pathophysiology of the various disorders, and the signs and tests which can be employed to discriminate between them. Discussions of medical treatment and other means of managing the vertigo are typically relegated to the final page or two of each chapter, and generally make up less than a tenth of the total text. This relative allocation of textbook space might suggest that although differential diagnosis of the nature of the dizziness is complex, once a correct diagnosis is achieved the treatment of the disease is uncomplicated. Unfortunately, only the first of these two premises is true. While the ambiguity of the symptoms and the multiplicity of the possible causes of vertigo and dizziness make diagnosis a very difficult task, the provision of effective treatment may not be possible even when the diagnosis is established. For example, Linstrom concludes, 'The task of the otolaryngologist, otologist, or neurotologist is not to make every dizzy patient well or even to diagnose the exact cause of imbalance in every patient. No one of us is capable of this' (1992: 745), while Browning notes that '[since] we cannot make a diagnosis with any degree of certainty in the majority of patients, management has to be empirical' (1991: 59). Thus while medical research continues to seek well-defined aetiologies and effective remedies, irremediable vertigo of uncertain origin remains a widespread complaint. Today's patients consequently often find themselves in a medical wilderness, void of definitive diagnoses and cures.

This state of affairs is not only disquieting for the patient, but also causes distinct unease amongst members of the medical profession. Indeed, the sections on vertigo in two recent textbooks on otolaryngology open with the candid admission that 'No other symptom strikes as much anxiety in the heart of the resident physician as the dizzy patient' (Katz 1986: 105), and 'Most otologists dread having to see a patient whose referral letter states that he has disequilibrium' (Browning 1986: 223). Similarly, Linstrom begins his comprehensive guide to 'Office management of the dizzy patient' with the observation that 'For many otolaryngologists, the management of a dizzy or vertiginous patient is an exercise in frustration' (1992: 745), while Wright introduces his guide for junior hospital doctors with the comment that 'having to diagnose and manage the dizzy patient may seem like being thrown in at the deep end when you can only just swim' (1988: 1).

When a patient first presents to the general practitioner with dizziness, the most parsimonious response of the doctor is to initiate a 'wait-and-see' policy, unless there are indications of a serious pathology, which can usually be identified quite readily from accompanying unmistakable signs of ear disease or of central neurological dysfunction (e.g. loss of consciousness, numbness or paralysis of the face or limbs, etc.). The practice of awaiting developments is logical, since doctors are aware that the most common forms of vertigo resolve spontaneously, and that those which do not are likely to be 'benign' (i.e. not life-threatening). Moreover, differential diagnosis of vertigo is based principally on the history of symptomatology over a period of time, while treatment is also largely a matter of trial and error. The initial response of the doctor to a complaint of vertigo therefore often consists of bland reassurance that the symptoms are not serious and will probably clear up. However, if the dizziness persists such reassurance is unlikely to be effective:

> You see you are told there is nothing wrong with you, then you get up the next day and feel exactly the same as you did. So it is all right being told, but if you are still feeling dizzy and having problems with your vision you can't accept what [the doctor] told you yesterday. You need to have something to work on.

Sometimes the lack of a firm diagnosis and absence of positive treatment is interpreted by patients as an indication that the doctor does not believe that the patient is really ill, or thinks that his or her symptoms are a sign of psychological disturbance. Many of the participants in my studies who had eventually received diagnoses of vestibular dysfunction felt that it had been difficult at first to convince their doctor that they were genuinely ill:

> They think you're putting the whole thing on, and you know you're not and it's so frustrating . . . You know how rotten you feel and you know how it affects you but you can't really get it over to them and then they're out to say 'What are you worried about?' You begin to wonder, 'Do they think I've got a problem?' and that's why you give up going back to the doctor.

> They [the doctors] thought it was just sort of agoraphobia, that when I got out and somebody took me out then it would be all right, but it wasn't – they wouldn't realise it was my balance as well. My doctor, at first, she just thought 'Oh well, she's just exaggerating' and then I got so bad that she really did realise that there was something wrong. I know a lot of it was anxiety, I was prepared to say that, OK, 80 per cent was anxiety, but the other 20 [per cent] was Ménière's because of the balance.

Doctors' views of vertiginous patients are indeed inevitably coloured by the awareness that dizziness is a common 'psychogenic' or 'non-organic' complaint, i.e. a symptom for which no physical explanation can be found, and which is believed to reflect underlying emotional problems. Specialists working in the field of otolaryngology are also likely to be familiar with the prevalent hypotheses regarding psychosomatic initiation or aggravation of organic vertigo mediated by anxious personality profiles and stress. Moreover, in many patients with organic vestibular disease, the absence of definitive signs of balance system dysfunction, coupled with the development of secondary anxiety and depression, can make their condition very difficult to distinguish from a psychological disorder. Similar diagnostic difficulties have, of course, been reported in the context of other disorders such as multiple sclerosis and AIDS (Goudsmit and Gadd 1991; Robinson 1988). However, the considerable overlap between symptoms of vertigo and of anxiety may render diagnosis of the organic origin of vertigo particularly problematic. Interestingly, the case of a woman whose vertigo (caused by Ménière's disease) was at first diagnosed as 'hysterical' illness is singled out by Roberts (1985) in her book on doctor–patient relationships, and is the only example she gives of a doctor mistaking physical disease for emotional distress.

In addition to the prevalence of psychogenic dizziness and the similarity between symptoms of anxiety and balance system dysfunction, there are two common psychological phenomena, which have been shown to affect interpersonal perception in a wide range of situations; they may also contribute to the tendency of doctors to suspect that patients complaining of dizziness are neurotic or emotional. The first is known as the 'actor–observer effect' (Watson 1982), because it can be attributed to the difference in perspectives between an observer and the person (the actor) who is the centre of the observer's attention. The actor looks outward towards the environment, and is therefore acutely aware of the changing situational factors which impact upon his or her attitudes and behaviour, whereas the observer focuses upon the actor and may not notice or fully register the importance of environmental influences. In the context of the doctor–patient relationship, the consequence is that the patient is conscious of the changing circumstances (in this case, a frightening and debilitating illness) which induce anxiety, whereas the doctor's attention is concentrated on the patient, who may appear to be an extremely agitated and distressed individual at the time of consultation. From my own experience, I can attest to the compelling nature of this perspective-induced perceptual bias; despite an intellectual conviction (based on intensive examination of the literature) that there is currently no sound evidence that people who develop vertigo are psychologically unstable before its onset, when attempting to reassure a succession of desperate and tearful patients I often find it difficult to imagine the same individuals as the confident and competent people that they were before they became ill, and as they are once more after recovery.

The second relevant cognitive process is the phenomenon of 'victim-blaming', which occurs in situations when one person feels powerless to alleviate the suffering of another (Gruman and Sloan 1983). Unable to accept the bleak and uncomfortable reality that the suffering of an innocent person cannot be prevented, most people unconsciously tend to rationalise the situation by supposing that the victim must be in some way responsible for his or her plight. It is clear from the preceding paragraphs that doctors feel particularly helpless when confronted with a complaint of persistent vertigo, and their own uncertainty and unease may sometimes unconsciously motivate them to dismiss their patients' problems as self-induced (by hypochondria or stress), or a sign of personal inadequacy (Hauser 1981).

Even when the physical origin of the symptoms is undeniable, doctors may be unwilling to discuss the diagnostic possibilities and prognosis in detail at an early stage. Although the genuine diagnostic and prognostic uncertainty make such reticence entirely comprehensible, the lack of information can leave the patients in an undesirable state of ignorance and apprehension, as the following accounts illustrate:

> The [company doctors] told me it was stress, so they sent me home. And the next day it happened, so it was happening every day . . . When they [colleagues] were carting me home from work they were just getting straight on the phone to [the company doctor]. He'd just come in, 'Oh, having one of these attacks again?' – but I didn't know what 'one of these attacks' were.

> I asked [the doctors] perhaps for something to be done and they say 'Well, you've just got vertigo, it's one of those things, a lot of people get it.'

> The duty doctor arrived about seven a.m. after I had been vomiting continuously since about one a.m. and his words to me were 'You've either got Ménière's disease or a tumour' and he walked out the door.

In many cases, patients with recurrent vertigo simply receive re-assurance from their local doctor that the vertigo is not a dangerous sign, sometimes coupled with trial or long-term prescriptions of a variety of drugs intended to limit or control the vertigo. Such treatment is presumably satisfactory or at least sufficient for many people, although no formal investigations have actually been carried out concerning levels of handicap, potentially remediable disability, or satisfaction with medical management amongst vertiginous patients who are not referred to a specialist. However, some people are unsatisfied with this state of uncertainty, and in their continuing quest for a diagnostic label, prognostic information and effective treatment they may seek a specialist opinion concerning their condition. The experiences of those referred to specialist clinics are considered in the following section.

UNDERGOING TESTING AND ACHIEVING A DIAGNOSIS

Referral to a specialist may be requested by the patient for the reasons given above, or may be considered appropriate by the general practitioner either because of a desire to exclude any possibility of a sinister cause, or because the patient exhibits relatively high levels of disability or distress. Patients referred to an otolaryngologist (i.e. ear, nose and throat, or ENT, specialist) or neurologist will be examined for signs of otological or neurological disease. Evidence of balance system dysfunction will also be sought, using tests of ocular control (such as the assessment of the control of eye movement when looking to right or left, or when following a moving object) and postural control (for example, the ability to stand heel-to-toe with eyes closed).

Significant central neurological dysfunction almost always leads to serious performance deficits on various tests of sensation and motor control, and the existence of central lesions can then be definitely confirmed or excluded by radiographic imaging (X-ray, CT scan or MRI scan). Similarly, the presence of active ear disease or injury can generally be quite easily determined by visual inspection and auditory testing, perhaps supplemented by surgical exploration. The most acute forms of vestibular dysfunction are also easy to recognise and confirm. On examination, the clinician can observe a distinctive pattern of eye movements ('nystagmus') which indicates disturbance of the vestibulo-ocular reflex, and if the sufferer is able to march on the spot with eyes closed, he or she will steadily turn in the direction of the damaged vestibular organ.

In many cases, however, the signs of balance system dysfunction are not so distinctive and definitive. Because of the natural process of compensation (described in the previous chapter), the manifest effects of balance system dysfunction caused by vestibular disorder are relatively brief, and their conspicuous influence upon the commonly performed activities used as clinical tests (such as standing still and looking to each side) often persists for no longer than a few days or weeks. Although latent vestibular-induced dysfunction may be detected by removing vision during these activities (so that the visual information cannot be used to compensate for distorted vestibular input), compensation frequently eliminates even these signs of vestibular imbalance during the many weeks or months that the patient may wait before requesting or obtaining an appointment with a specialist. Nevertheless, the individual may still be appreciably disabled when attempting more rapid or complex physical activities than those routinely tested in the clinic (see Chapter 3).

The clinical examination is usually supplemented by some specific tests of audiovestibular function. The most common are: (a) tests of hearing sensitivity (the 'audiogram'); (b) the positioning test, in which the patient is rapidly moved into various positions (including lying down) in order to examine the effect of head position on subjective sensations and eye movements; and (c) the caloric test, in which the vestibular organ in each ear can be independently stimulated by pouring warm and cool water into each ear canal in turn, thereby setting up thermal currents in the fluid in the inner ear which induce feelings of rotational movement and reflexive eye movements (nystagmus). However, abnormal audiovestibular test results are typically found in only a proportion of those patients whose clinical histories strongly suggest vestibular disorder (Yardley *et al.* 1992b). For example, examination of the test results of people who eventually developed unmistakable signs of Ménière's disease (progressive unilateral hearing loss and tinnitus plus severe episodic vertigo) revealed that only half had clear evidence of vestibular imbalance on caloric testing (Oosterveld 1979), and in the early stages less than half of such patients had the typical pattern of (low-frequency) hearing loss (Stahle *et al.* 1989). Moreover, even when abnormalities are found, these are relatively non-specific with respect to the underlying pathology. Hence, positional nystagmus may be associated with degeneration of the otoliths, viral infection, some deficiency of the blood supply to the inner ear, head injury, perilymph leak or endolymphatic hydrops (Baloh *et al.* 1987; Dix and Harrison 1984; Jongkees 1975; Oosterveld 1979). Similarly, vestibular imbalance revealed by the caloric test may be due to virtually any kind of disease or damage involving the inner ear or audiovestibular pathway. Moreover, while many signs of vestibular imbalance (particularly disordered vestibulo-ocular and postural reflexes) are transient, and disappear before the doctor has an opportunity to examine the patient, others (notably, an imbalance on the caloric test) persist indefinitely, and may be found long after compensation for the injury which originally caused the imbalance is achieved, and the patient has completely recovered. There is consequently little or no relationship between the subjective severity of symptoms and objective signs of vestibular dysfunction (Arenberg and Stahle 1980; Spitzer 1990; Yardley *et al.* 1992b).

The limited sensitivity of the basic tests may be augmented by a range of additional measures of hearing and balance function, including recording of auditory-evoked responses from the audiovestibular neural pathways, recording of eye movements induced by visual field motion or by rotation of the patient, and measurement of postural sway. However, no amalgamation of these techniques can yet provide a truly reliable and totally comprehensive evaluation of balance function. For example, even the optimal combination of results derived statistically from a fairly comprehensive test battery misclassified 36 per cent of the original classification sample of patients as normal, despite careful pre-selection of these patients on the basis of clear-cut, recent symptoms or signs of audiovestibular pathology (Allum *et al.* 1991). Similarly, in a review of 112 patients with a diagnosis of peripheral vestibular disorder, Voorhees (1989) noted that measurement of postural sway revealed dysfunction in 43 per cent of patients, comparing favourably with traditional tests of vestibulo-ocular function which were abnormal in only 28 per cent of patients. Although research into new diagnostic and functional tests continues, owing to the variety of pathologies and the differing rates of compensation for the diverse perceptual conditions and motor activities that the balance system must cope with, it is currently neither practicable nor even possible to identify the particular type of dysfunction of every patient.

Of course, when patients are sent by their doctors for specialist investigations they are unaware that the outcome may not entirely resolve their uncertainty. When the reason for referral is anxiety on the part of the patient or his or her local doctor about a possible sinister cause for their symptoms, the results of specialist testing may be awaited with a keen apprehension:

> I can't tell you what the anxiety was from week to week – not knowing what was wrong, and I was really ill.

Unfortunately, one of the consequences of the limitations of current tests of the balance system is that even after extensive testing, no clear indication of the cause of the vertigo may have been discovered. The doctors concerned will probably be fairly confident, after testing, that the vertigo is not caused by serious and active disease, but the complex details of whether and to what extent it is possible to exclude sinister pathology are not usually discussed with the patient. Warwick and Salkovskis (1985) have noted that, far from reassuring patients, referral for extensive investigations is frequently perceived by them as an indication that there is a real possibility that they may indeed be seriously ill. Consequently, when testing is inconclusive and the significance of the results is not explained in depth, the ignorance and anxiety experienced by patients may be exacerbated or prolonged, sometimes for years. This is illustrated by the following accounts, given by two patients whose examination and test results actually showed no evidence of sinister disease:

> When I first saw my doctor nothing was explained, and then I went to the hospital and nobody sat there and explained what was happening, why it was happening. Well, perhaps they didn't know, but you just go up to the hospital and they say, 'Right, we'll send you for some tests, take these tablets' and you don't know . . . nobody has said to me that I haven't got a tumour in my head, see nobody has said that, so there's slight concern still.

> [The consultant] put me through a CAT scan and a caloric test (which I vomited violently to), X-rays, hearing tests (my hearing is supposed to be fine). He put me through all these tests and he couldn't really say what it was, he couldn't give me an exact diagnosis . . . He said 'A couple of years and it should compensate.' So I waited a couple of years and it didn't compensate, so I went back to him . . . In all the tests put together I was slightly off the range – only by 1 per cent, 2 per cent in sort of worrying areas. Nobody would commit themselves 100 per cent and say 'You are OK,' which I wanted. I thought 'That is unfair, you have got the X-ray, you have got the CT scan, you can see if anything was lurking.' He would not tell me 100 per cent, and because I am a worrier I latched on to the fact he wouldn't tell me 100 per cent, so that exacerbated things and I came away feeling 'Nobody seems to be able to help me, they have washed their hands of me.'

This problem may be partly attributable to a failure in communication due to differences in the meanings that doctors and patients attach to customary medical phrases or styles of explanation. For example, when the doctor informs the patient that after extensive testing they could find nothing wrong, this message may be intended to convey reassurance that the potentially serious causes of the patient's illness have been excluded. However, the patient may interpret this information as meaning that the doctor has no idea what is causing the symptoms, which may therefore still signify some sinister, unidentified, and therefore untreated disease. Alternatively, the phrase may be taken to imply that the doctor doubts the organic basis of the symptoms, as one patient seemed to suspect:

> When I went back to speak to [the doctor] I would have liked him to have actually talked to me a lot more about it, and said you know there's nothing wrong there or there, but he just said 'Oh, they couldn't find anything, read this letter' and sort of smiled . . . It's very difficult, because I don't think I am at all the type of person to get het up, but when the doctor says that, you might not think you are but underneath you start to feel you are, so you've got to have a pretty strong mind to say no.

Stacey (1986) notes that if a health complaint is not legitimated by a medical diagnosis it cannot be attributed to external causes, and may instead be ascribed to attributes of the sufferer, such as their personality, age, gender or way of life. The preceding quotation certainly indicates that the failure to obtain a diagnosis may be viewed as an implicit accusation of personal inadequacy.

The provision of a diagnosis of vertigo due to peripheral vestibular dysfunction consequently brings relief from anxiety about sinister disease or accusations of malingering or emotional weakness:

> I was having all these tests, everything – heart, a brain scan – all of which showed absolutely nothing at all. My husband said to me 'Aren't you lucky you are so fit?' and I said, 'Why do I feel so awful?' That was before I came here [and was given a diagnosis of vestibular disorder]. I was pleased because at least I knew something was wrong, I mean it is much better than thinking that you are gradually going to deteriorate and not knowing the reason. It's pleasant to know that you've got an ear complaint and you've also got this dizziness problem and they're related. I feel a lot better to know that it's to do with my ear and balance than if it was to do with my heart.

> I was happy to find out that they had actually worked out what the problem was. Having gone on for nearly two years not knowing what the problem was, and people telling me 'There is nothing wrong with you' makes you wonder what is wrong. With being a balance problem one of the first things that came to mind was MS because my mother had that

– that was a worry, or possibly even a tumour of some sort. It was a relief to find out it was something relatively minor.

In his anthropological studies, Kleinman has identified 'cultural healing', which he defines as the 'provision of personal and social meaning for the experience of illness' (1986: 35), as a core function of any health care system. It is clear from the preceding quotations that a medical diagnosis plays a vital role in helping patients to make sense of their illness. Nevertheless, the significance of the test results and diagnosis must be carefully explained, as the following account given by a woman with advanced bilateral Ménière's disease illustrates:

> As part of the hospital treatment I had a balance test, when they shushed water into my ear, and [the doctors] told me I hadn't balance in my ears. And I was terrified then – they had told me initially I had no balance in one ear, and I thought, 'If it goes to the other side I'm going to be on my back for the rest of my life.'

This woman would have been spared considerable distress had she been told that orientation can be satisfactorily accomplished in most situations using vision and proprioception alone. The finding that she had virtually no vestibular function in either ear simply indicated that the disease had nearly run its course; although some problems with balance and ocular control would remain, the vertigo was likely to abate and she would certainly not be bedridden. Indeed, information is one of the most important aspects of care that the doctor can provide for people with vertigo, and will therefore be considered in greater detail in the final section of this chapter.

MEDICAL MANAGEMENT

Treatment of acute vertigo caused by vestibular dysfunction normally consists of symptomatic control by means of anti-emetics and drugs that partially suppress vestibular input. These drugs are not intended for long-term usage as they tend to retard natural compensation processes, and many have undesirable hypnotic properties (for a more detailed review of treatments for vertigo, see Chapter 6). Alternatively, or additionally, long-term prescription of antihistamines may be employed in an attempt to reduce the probability of further attacks. However, vertigo is a condition notoriously subject to placebo effects, spontaneous periods of remission, and unpredictable prognoses, and the true efficacy of preventative medication remains in question (Browning 1986; Dix

1984a). In cases of severe and intractable vertigo, an operation is sometimes suggested. The 'endolymphatic shunt' (or similar operation) may
be offered to patients with Ménière's disease, although in the only
clinical trial of this operation to include a placebo surgery group the
improvement apparently effected by the shunt operation was no greater
than the rate of placebo or spontaneous improvement (Thomsen *et al.*
1983). In cases of very severe vertigo, surgery to remove vestibular
input may be performed (Brackmann 1983). This is a fairly major
procedure; there may be permanent hearing loss on the operated side,
and many operations also involve a small risk of temporary facial palsy,
cerebrospinal fluid leak, or meningitis. In addition, the presence of
either bilateral disease or a failure of central compensation can render
the procedure ineffective.

Since there is no ideal treatment or panacea for vertigo, even after
extensive testing and the provision of the diagnosis the specialist may
well adopt the same empirical approach to management as that
employed by the local doctor:

> And [the consultant] will say 'Oh yes, you've got Ménière's disease
> and having problems with dizziness and that sort of thing . . . Um,
> come back and see me in six months.'

> It was vagueish, [the consultant] could not be precise as to what was
> the actual cause or what necessarily the actual problem was, but in
> common with the symptoms that it was likely to be vertigo and one
> of these three pills should have some effect. Unfortunately they
> didn't.

This outcome can be intensely disappointing to those individuals who
originally espoused what has been termed the 'mechanistic' model of
illness (Stainton-Rogers 1991), and believed that their symptoms were
the result of a discrete physical breakdown, which would be fixed by the
doctors once they had identified the cause:

> I wanted a magic cure I suppose – get rid of it, tablets for a week and
> then I am better.

> I was hoping they would just find out what it was and sort it out and
> have something to cure it – that was my idea.

Even people whose initial expectations concerning the outcome of
medical investigation and management were less optimistic may be
dismayed by the dearth of prognostic information which would allow
them to plan for and adapt to their condition:

The worst thing is not knowing how long it's going to last, and not knowing when the next one [attack] is going to come, and not knowing what I suppose the prognosis is – really, for me, I think it's the unknown.

In recognition of the profound disquiet that persistent vertigo can provoke, the main form of non-pharmacological support currently offered by the medical profession consists of 'reassurance'. The textbooks are unanimous in identifying reassurance of the patient as a key element of the medical management of vertigo, yet no specific advice as to how reassurance should be achieved appears to be considered necessary. In order to examine the effectiveness of routine reassurance, I used the statements about consequences and perceptions of vertigo made in interviews with patients as the basis for a questionnaire which was administered to all people with vertigo attending a specialist clinic in a one-year period. Although all of these patients had been thoroughly investigated, and reassured that their condition was 'benign' on at least two occasions by two different people, I found that two-thirds of the respondents admitted to continuing anxiety that something might be seriously wrong with them, and that this belief was highly correlated with reports of becoming depressed because of the vertigo (Yardley and Putman 1992).

The questionnaire also contained items relating to perceptions of treatment by medical staff. Previous studies of other types of illness have found that patients are generally unwilling to criticise medical care explicitly, but that dissatisfaction may be detected in the form of specific complaints, commonly concerning a perceived lack of information and interest in their problems, or the expressed belief that medicine has little to offer (Fitzpatrick 1984a; Roberts 1985; Thompson 1984). Responses to my questionnaire conformed precisely to this pattern; 81 per cent of respondents agreed to some extent that their doctors had been helpful, yet 70 per cent believed that nothing could be done for them. Many of the interviewees also tentatively suggested that more time and attention could have been devoted to discussion of their problems:

[The consultant] was very nice, but he tends to have his own idea as to what the cause of the problem is, and he doesn't listen. I suppose they've got so many patients – they have about five minutes before each patient to read through the notes and get their own idea of what the problem was. He didn't seem to really understand, he seemed to get the idea into his head that it was one thing and give me [vestibular sedatives, anti-emetics and antihistamines] – he couldn't think beyond that.

We do talk now, my doctor, but if we'd done it right from the start then I wouldn't have bothered him so much – that was one of my main problems. I do understand that perhaps there's not a lot known about the problem, why it happens, so I'm not blaming anybody you know, but that's the way I feel.

More detailed analysis of the questionnaire results revealed two distinct attitude profiles. Those who felt that they had benefited from drug treatment (and who had therefore presumably improved or recovered) stated that their doctors were helpful and understanding, and felt no desire for additional information and advice. However, half the sample agreed with the statement 'I wasn't given enough explanation of the illness and how to cope with it.' These people were characterised by elevated levels of reported handicap, disability, distress, and anxiety about the cause of the vertigo, and were less likely to consider their doctors helpful and understanding. These findings suggest that dissatisfaction with medical care may be the consequence of an awkward or belated transition from the traditional, doctor-centred mode of management which may be appropriate in cases of acute illness, to the co-operative style of doctor–patient relationship which is better suited to the management of chronic illness. Patients are quite content with minimal explanation and discussion if the problem of vertigo is quickly resolved, but the longer the symptoms persist and the more evident it becomes that there is no simple solution, the greater their desire for information which might help them to become actively involved in the management of their illness:

If there'd been something that actually said this is what's going on, this is the area of your body that's affected, this is what aggravates it, this is what can make it better, this is the drug therapy that's open to you, the different types of treatment available to you, this is what other sufferers have experienced, this is what they say about getting on with life – if that had been there, particularly if it had been written by somebody who'd actually been through it, I'm sure it would have been a help.

A further source of dissatisfaction described by many people concerned the hypothesised link between vertigo and stress. Because of the suspicion that psychological disturbance may be contributing to their patients' problems, doctors not infrequently mention that the vertigo may be stress-related. In the questionnaire study described above, virtually all the patients had diagnosed organic disease, but half the people in each diagnostic category responded positively to an item asking whether it had been suggested to them that stress might be a factor in their condition. Although this question did not specify whether the suggestion came from medical personnel, the interview statements on which it was based indicated that such suggestions most commonly originated from a medical source. Being told that the vertigo was stress-related was strongly associated with the complex of handicap, distress and dissatisfaction detailed above.

There are several possible explanations for this finding. Doctors may be particularly likely to proffer the suggestion that the vertigo is due to stress to patients whom they feel are unusually anxious. In addition, the failure of medical tests and treatments to provide a clear diagnosis and cure may simultaneously increase patients' anxiety and dissatisfaction with medicine, and doctors' suspicions of a non-organic contribution to their complaint. Alternatively, the mention of stress as a relevant factor may suggest to patients that their symptoms are thought to be exaggerated or neurotic and that their physical problem is therefore not fully appreciated, resulting in dissatisfaction with medical attitudes and care (Thompson 1984). Previous research has shown that reassurance is only effective when the patient feels that the doctor truly understands the nature of the complaint (Fitzpatrick 1984b); consequently, patients who believe (often rightly) that their symptoms have an organic cause are unlikely to accept 'reassurance' when accompanied by a comment that their symptoms may be stress-related. Indeed, those interviewees who had been told their vertigo was due to stress described three sources of anxiety: the original fear that there might be a sinister cause for symptoms that they knew to be real, coupled with the additional concern that the doctors believed them to be hypochondriac or neurotic, and a nagging doubt as to whether they might actually be so.

The management implications of the hypothesised link between vertigo and distress can be a further source of dissatisfaction. Since many psychoactive drugs are believed to also sedate the vestibular system, doctors not infrequently attempt to solve the suspected physical and psychological problems simultaneously by prescribing tranquillisers, phenothiazines, phenobarbitone, or other drugs with significant central effects. In this situation, the exact nature and purpose of the medication is seldom explained, and several patients in our sample were dismayed eventually to discover that the tablets they had been taking to prevent dizziness were tranquillisers. Such medication may have significant mentally *and* physically disorienting effects, as psychoactive drugs can disrupt balance system function and retard compensation (Ballantyne and Ajodhia 1984;

Pykkö *et al.* 1988). Since drugs of this kind are often habit-forming, there is also considerable potential for creating an indefinitely prolonged cycle of dizziness and drug dependence.

Some specialists go so far as to suggest surgical remedies for the anxiety experienced by people with vertigo. For example, Barber comments that 'fear of a recurrent vertigo . . . is a potent source of anxiety in some patients, and may constitute the main indication for surgical treatment' (1983: 29), while Browning follows a pessimistic evaluation of the probable physical value of surgery with the suggestion that 'the placebo effects of surgery should not be dismissed altogether, because it can be difficult to achieve similar placebo rates by non-surgical means' (1986: 240). However, the relative costs and benefits of these solutions have never been formally compared with any alternative non-surgical or non-pharmaceutical programme of management. The advisability, and indeed ethics, of deliberately addressing psychological problems by means of such techniques therefore deserves closer atten-tion, particularly since patients are typically not informed of the psycho-therapeutic rationale for these treatments, while both drugs and surgery carry the risk of undesirable side-effects.

Even when psychoactive medication is not prescribed, simply telling patients that their symptoms are stress-related can have negative psychosocial consequences, since formal attempts to help people suffer-ing from vertigo to identify, eliminate or cope with sources of stress (for example, by referral to a stress-management programme) are exceed-ingly rare. Many people perceive the mention of stress as a covert accusation that they are responsible for their illness, while the reaction of some is to assume that they should adopt the passive, restrictive life-style of a chronic invalid – a role which is itself a source of extreme frustration and stress for those who wish to be active. More often, patients attempt to find a sensible balance between activity and relaxa-tion, but feel hampered by uncertainty about the likely time-course of their symptoms and ignorance of how best to manage their disorder:

> You don't understand – is it going to go away, or is it something that you're always going to have, or is it something that will progress? You're never told that. I think right from the beginning it would have been really helpful to have been advised how to *cope* with it – not actually what's wrong with you or what it is. It's all very well being told to rest, but until you actually understand how to recognise when you are starting to have some problems . . . I think you have to almost, yourself, test yourself out – what you can and can't do.

As the preceding comments indicate, for many vertigo sufferers the final outcome of their medical career is the realisation that they will have to work out how to live with their illness themselves, often with little help from professional sources:

> In the end you become very philosophical about it because the impression you get is that nothing can be done about it anyway. I don't think the medical people knew, or still know nothing about it as far as I can see and they're really poking about in the dark, [so] in the end you don't bother people unless you're really desperate.

SUMMARY

This chapter has described how a disquieting degree of uncertainty accompanies every stage in the medical career of an individual with vertigo. Uncertainty about the cause and significance of symptoms of vertigo is frequently the principal reason for first consulting a doctor. Unfortunately, doctors are often unable to identify a definitive aetiology, owing to the difficulty of differential diagnosis and the limited sensitivity of clinical tests. One of the more distressing consequences of this diagnostic incertitude is that legitimation of the presence of an organic disorder may not be provided, and patients may feel that they are suspected of weakness of character or even malingering. Moreover, even if an organic disorder is confirmed, the prognosis for many forms of vertigo is unpredictable and there is no reliably effective form of medical treatment. The longer that symptoms persist, the greater the desire for information about what might cause, exacerbate or relieve the dizziness, but members of the medical profession sometimes appear unable or unwilling to discuss these questions in detail.

Eventually, people with chronic dizziness or vertigo come to realise that they will have to learn to live with the vagaries and complexities of their condition. The following chapters analyse the practical, physiological, social and psychological problems which confront people with chronic or recurrent vertigo, and describe the way in which people respond to these difficulties and learn to cope with the disorder.

Chapter 3

Physical activity and the environment

Vertigo and imbalance signal disruption to the perception and control of the physical orientation of the individual with respect to the environment. This chapter examines every aspect of that breakdown in the physical relationship between a person and his or her environment, from the dangers arising from loss of postural control to the phenomenological meaning of inability to maintain an upright posture.

The first section discusses disability – defined in this context as the limitation of physical activity by vertigo – and shows how the *anticipated* physical consequences of activity may lead to much greater disability than that imposed by actual physical incapacity. This section also details the potentially damaging physical and psychological effects of dizziness-induced disability.

In the second section, the nature of the disruption to perceptual-motor functioning is analysed. After exploring the evolutionary significance of the parallel syndromes of vertigo and motion sickness, an analysis of the factors which contribute to susceptibility and adaptation to motion sickness is undertaken, which identifies three important features of disorientation and imbalance. First, the nature of the situation that provokes disorientation can be quite specific, so that the same person may be markedly disorientated by one set of unusual or complex perceptual-motor conditions, but virtually unaffected by another. Second, it would appear that orientation is an active perceptual-motor achievement, and as such is affected by the experience, activities and skills of the individual concerned. Third, the degree of disability and malaise experienced by the individual seem to be determined chiefly by his or her ability to 'adapt', i.e. to develop the new modes of neuro-physiological and perceptual-motor functioning needed to overcome disorientation. The subsequent section therefore examines the processes and contextual factors which contribute to adaptation, comparing the acquisition of orienting skills in children, dancers, sailors, and people with vertigo.

The last section considers the way in which environmental conditions contribute to disorientation and imbalance; in particular, the phenomenon of 'visual vertigo', or disorientation provoked by situations characterised by unusual or impoverished visual information about self-motion. A critical review and integration of neuro- and psycho-pathological accounts of visual vertigo forms the basis for an explanation of how perceptual factors and rational fears may combine to produce disorientation and anxiety in challenging perceptual environments. Finally, the psychosocial consequences of this change in the relationship with the environment are described.

PHYSICAL CONSEQUENCES OF VERTIGO

The physical characteristics of vertigo (detailed in Chapter 1) comprise, first, the disorientation and loss of postural and ocular control that characterises balance system dysfunction and, second, the ancillary autonomic symptoms such as cold sweating, nausea and vomiting, which are triggered by perceptual disorientation. The immediate physical consequence of an acute attack is therefore virtual incapacity. The sufferer cannot stand or walk and may not even be able to focus properly owing to involuntary eye movements, and must therefore simply lie still in bed, avoiding any head movements which might stimulate the vestibular system and thus exacerbate the dizziness. Since the process of compensation is quite rapid, this state of extreme disability rarely lasts for more than an hour or two, but symptoms sufficiently severe to confine the individual to bed may continue for a day or two. Thereafter, until complete habituation is achieved, any rapid or unaccustomed movement will provoke further symptoms, resulting in a less extreme but nevertheless significant degree of discomfort and interference with physical activity.

The far-reaching effects of residual, movement-provoked vertigo on physical activity are graphically described in the following quotations:

> If I get up very quickly I get it [vertigo], if I bend down I get it, if I bend, if I stretch, if I look up it starts me up, if I turn I get giddy – I can't turn that side.

> I get out of bed very slowly, like a zombie. I've learned not to bend and not to turn quickly. I never look at my feet – if I drop things I wouldn't dream of bending down to pick it up.

It is evident from these reports of significant disability that recurring vertigo is not simply an unpleasant experience, but can have an extensive impact on various areas of normal activity. Many people find that turning or tilting the head, or bending backwards or forwards, can provoke vertigo. This inevitably causes problems with such routine chores as cleaning and tidying, digging and lifting, transferring shopping to and from trolleys, or even washing their hair. Difficulty in focusing the eyes sometimes affects pastimes such as reading, knitting and sewing. Persistent unsteadiness or the possibility of a sudden unexpected attack renders some tasks too risky or responsible to be undertaken; in a study of handicap associated with recurrent vertigo (Yardley et al. 1992c) the majority of those interviewed had been obliged to give up driving, and some reported being unable to operate machinery, supervise children, cycle, or swim. A common experience is that susceptibility to travel sickness is greatly increased (see following sections), to the extent that it may be difficult to cope with even the passive travel involved in long business trips or holidays. In addition, many physical leisure pursuits, such as dancing, sport or exercise, may induce such disagreeable sensations of imbalance and nausea that they no longer seem worth pursuing.

From the explanations given by sufferers for the various instances of disability, it appears that although some of the disability caused by vertigo is the direct result of loss of postural or ocular control and general malaise, much of the restriction of activity is not due to current physical incapacity. Indeed, when the extent of the handicap resulting from vertigo is compared with the frequency and severity of symptoms, it is clear that quite limited and isolated episodes of dizziness may nevertheless be associated with prolonged and substantial restrictions on life-style (Yardley et al. 1994a). The apparent discrepancy between the incidence and degree of physical incapacity and the consequent disability can be explained in terms of the rational response of sufferers to symptoms provoked by movement, which is to avoid any activities which seem to trigger vertigo. Such deliberate restriction of activity has been termed 'anticipatory disability' (Cioffi 1991).

Anticipatory disability is sometimes ascribed to a fearful or passive mode of responding to physical ailments. This interpretation of self-imposed restrictions on life-style might seem justified when the sole purpose is to avoid provoking sensations that the sufferer finds unpleasant – for example, when people with vertigo restrict their movements simply in order to avoid provoking disagreeable symptoms. However, the unpredictability and uncertainty surrounding vertigo provide two further compelling reasons why even the most stoic and energetic of individuals might think it best to avoid activity. First, an important rationale for restricting physical movement emanates from the suspicion or belief that, since movement is unmistakably linked to the onset of sensations of dizziness, immoderate levels of activity could trigger a full-scale attack. The following accounts clearly demonstrate that sufferers find it difficult to distinguish between dizziness induced by head movement and the initial stages of an acute episode of vertigo:

> I would feel light-headed if I was bending down, dress-making or anything like that (I tend to do it on the floor). It would tend to make me feel a little bit dizzy, which would sometimes trigger off a dizzy attack.

> I have to be ever so careful how I move and what I do. Every time I bend my head down I have this really awful giddy head – last time I went to the Bingo I had to sort of sit and hold my head still while I try and mark off the numbers . . . I went into the DIY shops, and I had to come out because it was making me sick sort of going around looking at things and sort of moving my head around. The movement of my head seemed to – I don't know whether that's what set it off, but that's what it appeared. Even now, if I have to turn round quick and then have to turn back again, I feel that it's going to come on.

The (essentially erroneous) belief that movement might be the underlying cause of acute attacks of vertigo is sometimes regarded as a rationale for espousing complete immobility as a logical preventative or coping strategy:

> I suppose if you were clever enough just to go to bed, lay down twenty-four hours before the attack really materialised you might have been able to stabilise it that way.

> I mean I haven't been doing *anything*, full-stop. Whether or not it is just complete rest [that is needed] I don't know. I mean, not working, just sitting in a chair doing what you want all day, whether or not that is giving the body rest, time to recuperate I don't know, I have got no idea. All I know is I am not getting up, the usual routine, and going out to work, tearing back and cooking a meal and all that goes with it.

These quotations illustrate the immense potential for anticipatory disability which can result from ignorance of the distinction between spontaneous attacks, which are caused by internal damage to the vestibular organ and are quite unrelated to activity, and the movement-provoked vertigo which constitutes a necessary and harmless, albeit

disagreeable, part of the process of compensation. Although the symptoms provoked by movement are indeed very similar to those experienced during a mild spontaneous attack, awareness of the entirely
different causes and implications of spontaneous and provoked disorientation would permit sufferers to regulate their activity levels in a
more informed and appropriate manner.

A second motivation for refraining from certain activities is the, often
very real, possibility of causing harm to oneself or to others whilst
incapacitated; examples of actual mishap given by the interviewees
included staggering into furniture, tripping over, and even falling under
a lorry. Since many people find that an attack can occur at any time,
virtually without warning, a prudent strategy is to avoid all activities
which could prove dangerous if disrupted by sudden dizziness. Driving
is the most commonly reported instance of an activity of this kind,
although people with vertigo often conclude that the handicapping
consequences of giving up driving would be so severe that they prefer
to trust that they would be able to stop the car safely when an attack
began. However, many other activities may be considered too
dangerous to undertake, from scaffolding to stage-lighting, and from
crossing roads to climbing stairs.

The extent to which vertigo represents a potential danger varies
according to the activities the individual is typically engaged in; hence,
people who are required by their occupations to scale heights or operate
dangerous machinery are more handicapped by vertigo than those who
have office jobs. The threat posed by vertigo also depends upon the
physical resources that the individual is able to call upon to prevent or
to cope with the possibility of falling. This could partly explain why
increasing age has been shown to augment the level of disability resulting from vertigo (Yardley *et al.* 1992d). Even a mild vestibular lesion
may cause significant disruption to postural control in people with
multiple minor sensory or motor impairments (as is often the case in the
elderly). They may be unable to substitute or correct for absent or
altered vestibular information owing to poor vision or reduced somatosensory function in the lower limbs. Moreover, because they have
generally slower reflexes, reduced joint mobility and less muscular
strength, older people are less able to correct their posture once they
have begun to overbalance (Lee 1989). In addition, not only do older
individuals find it more difficult to accommodate or compensate for a
partial, momentary loss of equilibrium, but they may also find the
physical consequences of an actual fall are more damaging, owing to
brittle bones and reduced recuperative powers.

Vertigo can cause secondary physical harm not only by inducing falls, but also as the result of the physical strategies adopted to prevent or cope with dizziness. One of the most common side-effects of attempting to avoid head movement is the development of a stiff neck, which can also lead to severe headache. Often sufferers are quite unaware that they have unconsciously adopted a rigid head posture, and assume that the headaches are simply an integral part of the syndrome of dizziness, nausea and general malaise. Ironically, cervical (neck) disorder is itself believed by many clinicians to cause dizziness, either by distorting the somatosensory input from the neck or by disrupting the vascular supply to the inner ear (de Jong and Bles 1986; Oosterveld 1984; Pfaltz 1984). Although cervical disorders may be caused by spontaneous degeneration or disease, they may also be exacerbated by deliberately maintaining an overly rigid head posture (Beyts 1987; Ödkvist and Ödkvist 1988). Hence, by employing a stiff upright head posture to cope with residual dizziness due to a vestibular disorder, people with vertigo may actually compound the causes of their dizziness. In addition, a general loss of fitness and mobility, sometimes accompanied by weight gain, is a common long-term effect of the restriction of physical activity associated with chronic vertigo, since sufferers generally abandon all forms of sport and vigorous exercise.

The consequences of restricting head and body movement have social as well as physical dimensions. Mauss (1979) notes that there are socially specific modes of performing any physical movement, which will vary according to the social characteristics of the individual, such as their culture, age and status. Posture and head movement constitute an important non-verbal channel of communication, which can convey attitudes such as interest, dominance or assent. The postural strategies used to cope with vertigo can affect the non-verbal element of social relations in subtle but important ways:

> You don't look at somebody who approaches you from the right hand side, you wait until they get right round before you talk to them. If anyone's talking to me, I would mostly stand up and talk to them, I wouldn't look up at them.

Toombs (1992) has pointed out that, in social terms, the body can be considered as a meaningful gestural display. In this respect, people who change their behaviour as a result of vertigo may be concerned about the negative impression that their physical caution might make on observers:

People might say 'Run along the road, jump in the air, do all sorts of things', but I won't do those things. I am unfit anyway, but I am frightened of bringing on an attack. Running around, mucking about, being playful really – you know, anything like that I am very wary of . . . these elaborate fairs they have now, lots of things I will avoid. It does put a dampener, you know, if you want to be a fun person.

I take a little bit longer about everything; people will say that's age, but it isn't age, it's because I'm frightened of falling over.

The somewhat defensive tone of these quotations suggests that the unflattering perceptions attributed to observers, such as slowness and lack of spontaneity, may be partly internalised, resulting in a negative body-image or even self-image.

Toombs also observes that under normal circumstances we are unaware of our body, which simply constitutes the means employed for the purpose of activity. Only when activity is disrupted by physical malfunction does the body become the focus of our attention, and in this context it is perceived as defective, and in opposition to the self. Some of the comments made by people with vertigo confirm that sudden disorientation and loss of control can induce an alienating awareness of one's own body:

You could be all right one moment and then it's like throwing a switch, and you feel quite ill – not ill, you become very tense and very introspective of yourself, almost as if there'd been a chemical switch in your body.

I reckon it hits you a bit like having a close death in the family; your body has been changed, it's out of your hands – part of you is not the same, will never be the same again.

In sum, the physical consequences of vertigo, while unpleasant and frustrating in themselves, can have much more profound implications through their indirect psychosocial impact. Restrictions on activities such as driving and physical exertion, adopted either out of necessity or concern about physical danger, or motivated by fear of provoking attacks, may force some individuals to give up work and impose limitations on the independence and social activities of many others. Similarly, abandoning active leisure pursuits, such as dancing or rambling, can cause a range of adverse secondary effects, from becoming fat and unfit to losing contact with valued social networks. The result may be a self-image of apparent premature ageing, as the individual finds him- or herself confined to moving stiffly and cautiously around the home. The multiple ways in which physical disability caused by vertigo can lead to further physical problems, social difficulties and psychological distress are eloquently exemplified in the reply of one young woman to the question 'In what way is vertigo affecting your life?':

> Well, it obviously affects pleasure, all aspects of pleasure. You know, I need to exercise for fitness. There are things I want to do just for my reasons. Sex it affects – you try to romp around the bed with somebody. So what it has done is has affected my sex life like anything, because I am too frightened of getting dizzy, so I will avoid it. It has affected my work in the sense that I will get somebody else to do something rather than me, like bend down or do this, that and the other – I feel guilty about it because it is unfair. The travelling; I panic if I have to get in a car and sit at the back seat, so I push and bully to get in the front seat. And anything that would really trigger it – sitting upright in the morning I get out of bed very slowly. This makes me feel like an old person, which is awful, I feel very old and decrepit. I try not to turn round suddenly – I feel like I have got a brace around my neck most of the time. I wake up with these stiff necks a lot of mornings, and I think 'Why is this?' and I am sure some of this is worry and tension, and I think it is the fact that I am walking around continuously like I am a Munster [a stiffly-moving zombie character on television].

PARALLELS WITH MOTION SICKNESS

In the preceding section, attention was focused on the bodily consequences of vertigo and the way in which the physical activities of the individual affect and are affected by vertigo. However, disorientation is not an internal somatic sensation, located entirely within the body, but an awareness of a disturbed relationship with the environment. Indeed, vertigo is frequently described by sufferers in terms of an uncertain orientation with respect to the environment, or is explicitly portrayed as an alarming motion of the environment itself:

> Sometimes you don't know which way up you are – it's really strange.

> Every time I looked up the room used to spin round, the whole ceiling just spun.

> One time I was watching television and the television was going round and round, the whole set appeared to go round and round. If

you shut your eyes everything would still go round and round, so it was frightening in that respect.

These phenomenological accounts depict the experience of vertigo as arising at the interface between the individual and the surroundings, rather than within the individual. It is certainly the case that equilibrium demands co-ordination between the individual and environment; physical activity must be accurately calibrated to match external conditions. Hence, in the same way that a change in the usual pattern of signals from the vestibular organ can result in vertigo, unfamiliar or altered environmental conditions can also cause disorientation, imbalance and sickness. Some clinicians have therefore suggested that motion sickness can be regarded as a special case of vertigo (Brandt and Daroff 1979), since the symptoms of motion sickness and vertigo are very similar, and a comparable pattern of gradual adaptation mediates recovery from both forms of disorientation. The correspondence between the subjective experience of disorientation caused by internal and external conditions is also recognised by people who have experienced both, as a former aviator explained:

> It [the onset of vertigo] stopped me from wanting to fly. I used to like plane loop-the-loops and all those sort of things when I was younger, and I was going to start to take it up again, but I decided that vertigo was quite a sufficient sensation by itself – you've got your own personal simulator!

An appreciation of the parallels between vertigo and motion sickness is important for two reasons. First, an understanding of their shared aetiology may provide clues to the essential functional origin, nature and purpose of the syndrome. Second, by analysing the principles governing responses to disorientation in people with normally functioning balance systems (i.e. motion sickness) it may be possible to obtain insights into the processes involved in disorientation caused by balance system dysfunction. The following subsections therefore examine the fundamental basis for motion sickness and vertigo, and the key features of perceptual-motor responses to disorientation.

The evolutionary significance of vertigo and motion sickness

Motion sickness and vertigo both appear to be triggered solely by disorientation involving the vestibular system. For example, when disruption to orientation and balance is due to disorders which result in peripheral somatosensory dysfunction or loss of motor control (e.g. numb or paralysed legs), no dizziness or nausea is provoked. Similarly, the only people who are completely resistant to motion sickness under all circumstances are those who have no functioning vestibular system (Money 1990). It therefore seems possible that the evolutionary purpose of the syndrome of vertigo and motion sickness is specifically to alert the animal or human concerned to a balance system dysfunction caused by vestibular failure, and to promote appropriate behavioural responses (chiefly, immobility while dangerously uncoordinated) and physiological reactions (such as vomiting, to expel any poisonous substance which may have caused the dysfunction).

Deficiencies in perception or motor control caused by other types of sensory or motor dysfunction can be signalled by modality-specific, localised symptoms such as pain, numbness, weakness, loss of sensation, blurring or blindness. However, the vestibular system has evolved in such a way that it functions only in conjunction with other sensory and motor systems, and on its own yields no distinct sensations. Therefore, a dysfunction of the vestibular system can *only* be identified indirectly. Vertigo or motion sickness consequently ensues whenever a persistent breakdown in perceptual co-ordination and control of orientation occurs for which no other obvious internal or external cause can be detected, hence signalling a probable disruption of vestibular functioning. This is why the syndrome is not provoked by orientation difficulties due to darkness or blindness, or the co-ordination problems caused by entering a new medium such as water, or attempting to maintain balance during a new mode of locomotion, such as skiing or cycling; in these situations the cause of the balance problems is easily perceived. In contrast, although the fact of disorientation due either to vestibular dysfunction or to sea or space travel is apparent, the ambiguities in the peripheral information which result in disorientation in these situations are certainly not immediately obvious to the individual concerned.

Before the invention of the passive modes of transport and artificial environments which nowadays provoke sickness, any prolonged alteration in the way in which a human needed to interact perceptually with the environment for the purposes of orientation was likely to be due to vestibular dysfunction. Moreover, because of the adaptable nature of the orientation system, awareness of inexplicable disorientation provides a particularly suitable means of alerting the individual to vestibular dysfunction. Clearly, what is important to an active person is his or her state of co-ordination, rather than the absolute level of vestibular functioning.

This information can be provided by a syndrome which is provoked indirectly, through the awareness of disorientation. The extremely variable pattern and time-course of adaptation which characterises recovery from vertigo is, by this mechanism, precisely shadowed by symptoms of vertigo; consequently, these symptoms provide the individual with an up-to-date index of his or her level of co-ordination.

Principles derived from the study of motion sickness

Recognition of the close parallels between vertigo and motion sickness can provide valuable information about the way in which both activity and environment may affect people with disorientation. The study of clinical vertigo is complicated by variations in pathology, which cannot be accurately assessed, and secondary adaptations to chronic balance problems. In contrast, motion sickness can be provoked in controllable, isolated episodes, using standardised stimuli, allowing *normal* responses to challenges to the orientation system to be examined. By drawing upon experimental studies of motion sickness it is therefore possible to derive insights into vertigo which would be difficult to obtain by means of investigations set in the context of naturally occurring pathology and the multifaceted, uncontrolled experiences of patients. Principles governing provocation of motion sickness and adaptation to disorientation in healthy people can then be extended to the case of those suffering from vertigo. Three important conclusions derived from a review of the copious studies of motion sickness are presented below (for a detailed analysis of motion sickness, see Yardley 1991a, 1992).

Situation-specific disorientation

The first principle that can be deduced from research into motion sickness is that an individual's reactions to disorienting conditions are partly situation-specific. For example, people who are quite disoriented by the vertical motion of waves may be completely undisturbed when spun around in a rotating chair. This finding has obvious implications for evaluation of balance system dysfunction; accurate assessment of disability is more likely to be achieved under test conditions which differ as little as possible from the circumstances that the individual finds disorienting in everyday life. This may partly explain why the results of the traditional tests of vestibular function, which chiefly involve measuring the eye movements of an inactive patient in the dark, often yield negative results in patients with symptoms which nevertheless strongly suggest balance system dysfunction. The fact that disorientation may be experienced only in certain situations or when performing particular orientation tasks is appreciated by clinicians such as Norré, who recommends multiple assessments of compensation for vestibular dysfunction, including evaluation of nystagmus and vertigo resulting from position, movement, visual stimuli, and rotation (at several different frequencies), and postural instability under various conditions (Norré 1988; Norré et al. 1984). Norré has observed that a patient may display no evidence of functional abnormality when rotated at low speeds, whereas high speed rotation may produce clear signs of a failure to adapt to vestibular imbalance (or vice versa). Similarly, the pace and stage of adaptation of the vestibulo-ocular reflex can be markedly dissociated from compensation in terms of vestibular control of posture. Someone who has completely normal eye movements may therefore still experience difficulty in balancing. In addition, dysfunction may be apparent *only* under particular perceptual conditions; for example, when visual cues for orientation are unusual or misleading (see subsection on 'visual vertigo' in this chapter).

The influence of perceptual-motor experience, skills and activities

A second principle that can be inferred from research into disorientation is that the perceptual-motor experience, skills and activities of people can affect their reactions to a potentially disorienting environment. Experience of disorienting conditions may result in the development of appropriate perceptual-motor strategies for actively coping with them (such as the methods used by dancers to overcome dizziness, described in the following section). One instance is the observation by Fukuda (1975) that bus drivers lean in the opposite direction to passengers when navigating a bend; such postural strategies may well be relevant to the observation that people are typically more resistant to motion sickness while actively engaged in driving a vehicle than when they are passive passengers (Benson 1984). On the other hand, perceptual 'habits' learned in one environment may prove maladaptive in some situations. For example, experienced pilots, who have a keen appreciation of the patterns of perceptual information to be expected in flight, actually become *more* disoriented (and sick) in flight simulators than do novice pilots (Crowley 1987). The 'cabin' environment seems to specify the perceptual conditions pertaining during flight and therefore cues the use of orientation information appropriate to flying, but actually the perceptual information in a simulator is not quite the same as in a real aeroplane.

In clinical terms this implies that, in addition to assessing the basic input from each sensory system, it is essential to consider the way in which the individual actively attends to and combines these signals. For example, after a transient vestibular disorder many people fully recover the vestibular input they temporarily lost, but experience continued imbalance. Often these individuals have normal vestibular responses to tests of vestibulo-ocular function, but do not appear to use vestibular information for postural control (Black *et al.* 1989); presumably they automatically adjust to the initial disorder by subconsciously ignoring or suppressing the distorted vestibular input, but then fail to abandon this perceptual strategy even if the vestibular information is once again accurate and useful (Black and Nashner 1984a, 1984b). Since the utilisation of perceptual information depends upon the characteristics and activities of the individual concerned, these can strongly influence the resulting degree and form of functional disability. This may further explain the limited ability of clinical tests to predict disorientation in everyday situations; whereas the clinical vestibular tests assess the semi-automatic reflexes of patients passively exposed to vestibular stimulation, vertigo in everyday life may either be prevented or provoked by the perceptual-motor strategies used by these individuals to cope with a variety of environments. New tests are already being developed to supplement the traditional vestibular test battery by providing a more complete and naturalistic assessment of orientation system function or disability, and for monitoring the state of compensation the patient has achieved. Examples include the measurement of eye movements induced by rotation at a wide range of frequencies (Cyr *et al.* 1989) or by actively and rapidly shaking the head (Takahashi *et al.* 1990), evaluation of the way in which patients use visual, vestibular and somatosensory information for postural control (Nashner *et al.* 1982), and the ability of people with vestibular deficiencies to judge the distance they are turned in the dark (Brookes *et al.* 1993).

The importance of adaptation

The third conclusion that can be derived from the literature on motion sickness is that, at least in healthy people, the degree of malaise provoked by disorienting conditions seems to depend less on their immediate reactions than on their ability to adapt to these conditions. Research has revealed reliable differences between individuals in their rate, retention and transfer of protective adaptation to disorienting situations (Graybiel and Lackner 1980). It therefore seems likely that people will also differ in their rate of adaptation after a vestibular disorder, and their susceptibility to the disinhibition of habituation which may be responsible for recurrences of dizziness in the absence of new or progressive organic disorder. (A further logical deduction is that people who have a history of motion sickness may be slow to adapt to a change in balance system function, although this hypothesis has never been formally, and prospectively, tested.) Hence, whereas the number and severity of spontaneous vertiginous attacks is determined by pathology, individual differences in the persistence of malaise and disability may be determined principally by the ability to adapt – or, in clinical terms, to compensate. This conclusion acquires particular significance in the light of the evidence, detailed in the following chapters, suggesting that the emotional distress often felt by people with vertigo is more closely related to chronic disability and handicap than to the frequency and severity of episodes of acute disorientation. The processes involved in adapting to disorientation therefore deserve more careful consideration.

ADAPTATION AND LEARNING

There are several different, albeit probably interrelated, forms of adaptation to disorientation, ranging from central neurological 're-programming' of the way in which particular patterns of sensory input are combined for orientation, to the development of flexible perceptual-motor strategies and skills.

Immediate adaptation following an acute vestibular episode appears to proceed partly by means of some semi-automatic neurological processes; for example, in order to reduce the vestibular imbalance, vestibular signals from the healthy vestibular organ may be partially suppressed by the central nervous system for several weeks. Longer-term compensation for vestibular impairment involves a process sometimes referred to as 'central recalibration', whereby the balance system adjusts to the new pattern of sensory information which now accompanies each head movement (see Chapter 1). By means of central recalibration the orientation system gradually attains a new equilibrium, which is manifested at the neurological level as recovery of vestibular-related activity at the level of the brain-stem (i.e. in the vestibular nuclei of the impaired vestibular system), despite permanent damage to the peripheral vestibular organ. The progressive supplementation or replacement of lost vestibular information by information from the healthy vestibular sensors and the visual and somatosensory systems occurs as the result of repeated experience of movement. Consequently, the 'recalibration' element of habituation is quite movement- and situation-specific; only those combinations of sensory input that are experienced many times cease to provoke disorientation and sickness. The implication is that any unaccustomed movement or environment will continue to cause difficulties; although vertigo may not be induced by routine activities, a twist of the head performed more quickly than usual or a trip on a ferry may unexpectedly cause renewed dizziness and nausea.

Research into motion sickness suggests that in addition to this principal, localised form of habituation it is possible to acquire a degree of general resistance to disorientation. One example of this is the fairly substantial transfer of adaptation from a certain motion to a set of similar motions. For instance, experiments have shown that habituation developed while being rotated in a chair in one direction transfers to some extent to rotation in the opposite direction, and adaptation to precise left–right or fore–aft head movements performed while rotating generalises to multidirectional head movements (Reason and Brand 1975). This kind of habituation transfer provides the rationale for treatment programmes designed to provide protective adaptation for chronically motion-sick aviators (e.g. Stott 1990). Such programmes often employ exposure to a highly circumscribed set of activities and perceptual conditions, such as performing stereotyped head movements in a rotating chair, to increase tolerance of the much more diverse and complex activities and perceptual conditions which provoke sickness during flight.

A general resistance to disorientation is often seen in people whose occupations involve repeated exposure to unusual motion, such as sailors, pilots, and athletes (Bles and van Raay 1988; Crémieux and Mesure 1990; Dowd and Cramer 1971). Dancers and skaters provide a particularly instructive example of generalised resistance to orientation. Dancers are less influenced than most people by misleading visual information about the location of their body parts provided by distorting prisms, and are able to retain a relatively precise sense of their position (Kahane and Auerbach 1973). They are also able to suppress most of the compensatory eye movements, imbalance, and feelings of rotation (and nausea), that are normally induced by rotatory and caloric tests, even though these tests differ considerably in terms of motor commands and sensory input from actively pirouetting about an earth-vertical axis (McCabe 1960). This resistance to the effects of motion is acquired; McCabe was able to chart the development of suppression of rotatory and caloric responses in skaters as they learned to spin.

Close examination of how dancers react to passive rotation suggests that many different kinds of perceptual strategy or sensorimotor learning may mediate their resistance to its effects. For example, all dancers learn the technique of 'spotting', which consists of breaking up the constant rotation into shorter bursts of motion by keeping the head still for most of the turn and then whipping it around. This technique also requires learning to attend to useful visual information by means of 'fixation', which simply involves staring at a stationary object in order to prevent reflexive eye movements and provide a stable reference point for orientation. Fixation is a strategy which many people report that they spontaneously use to cope with attacks of vertigo (Austin 1992). However, even when such techniques are prohibited, dancers tend to be more resistant than normal to the effects of rotation, but they each seem to develop differing kinds of resistance. For example, some can suppress the compensatory eye movements almost completely even in the dark, when optic fixation is not possible, while others show a normal, vigorous pattern of eye movements in response to rotation (Osterhammel et al. 1968). Nevertheless, the two essential adaptive responses to rotation that they all share are that after a spin they can balance well, and feel no dizziness at all.

The phenomenon of partial generalisation of adaptation is, to some extent, already exploited to the benefit of vertiginous patients in the form of exercise-based rehabilitation, which encourages patients to engage in a subset of all possible eye, head, and body movements in order to develop sensorimotor co-ordination anew. The rationale for this form of rehabilitation is hence very similar to the logic justifying motion sickness prevention programmes for aviators which employ habituation to a limited range of activities and motions. Some more sophisticated rehabilitation programmes are also starting to address the specific problems that may be caused by particular perceptual and motor strategies (for a more extensive discussion, see Chapter 6). In view of the partly situation-specific nature of disorientation, it seems reasonable to argue that rehabilitation should also include practice in orienting in the actual situations causing disorientation in everyday life – in the same way that, in the treatment of chronically sick aircrew, adaptation to provocative motions in the laboratory is routinely supplemented with graded exposure to actual flight (Stott and Bagshaw 1984). In addition, the resistance to disorientation generally seen in people such as dancers, gymnasts, sailors and pilots suggests that by regularly undertaking difficult balancing tasks, or confronting challenging orientation environments, it may be possible to develop a degree of valuable perceptual-motor 'fitness' or skill, in the same way that aerobic exercise can help to maintain optimal cardiovascular functioning.

Effects of context on the process of acquiring orientation skills

Since it would appear that the achievement of co-ordinated orientation and balance can be considered an acquired perceptual-motor skill, it is interesting to examine the factors which encourage and support the development of skilled co-ordination, and those which may hinder or obstruct the attempts of people with vertigo to relearn orientation skills and capabilities. The physical and sociocultural context of the disorientation may play an important role in this respect, in so far as it constrains the availability of suitable opportunities for learning orientation skills and shapes expectations concerning the possibility of overcoming disorientation and the appropriateness of various behavioural responses to dizziness and imbalance.

In the past, when humans were obliged to hunt for meat, run for safety, and stoop or climb to obtain roots, fruit, water and shelter, the inescapable activities of daily living would probably have been sufficient to ensure rapid and thorough compensation after a balance system disorder. However, in modern society the conditions for perceptual-motor learning may be less favourable for adults than for children, who exhibit an attraction to disorienting activities which contrasts with the marked aversion to activities provoking dizziness displayed by most vertiginous adults. Simple observation reveals that children are naturally inclined to explore the limits of their environment and their orientation skills; toddlers delight in being spun, tossed or turned upside down, older children go out of their way to balance on high walls, perform handstands and somersaults, and ride on terrifying helter-skelters. Social structures strongly support these activities; every playground incorporates swings and roundabouts, and gymnastics is a part of the formal educational curriculum. The example set by both parents and peers also encourages persistence despite initial fears, or indeed motion sickness, which are viewed simply as a natural phase to be overcome, rather than an insuperable obstacle. In consequence, the child passes beyond the initial stage of disorientation, and acquires the perceptual schemata which are required in order to utilise appropriately the information pertaining to each special environment, and the action schemata which support skilled and co-ordinated activity within them.

Adults are much less likely to seek out these types of learning experience, and have limited access to situations and social roles which permit exploration of the boundaries of orientation. Any adult spotted swinging around a lamppost or walking precariously along a narrow wall would be considered juvenile, if not actually mentally disordered.

The most plausible role model for the vertiginous individual to adopt is that of a partial invalid, who would be considered foolhardy to persist in activities that apparently exacerbated a medical condition. Moreover, the safe and structured learning situations of the child are not a natural part of the environment of the adult, who may have to struggle to master disorientation while driving, negotiating a business deal, or clambering around scaffolding with no safety harness. To an adult, disorientation in a certain environment or during a particular activity is therefore seen not as a learning phase, but as an unnatural and embarrassing sign of disability. These factors help to explain why an adult may rapidly come to perceive activities or environments which provoke disorientation simply as a source of physical and social discomfort, rather than a pleasurable opportunity to investigate the possibilities for co-ordination and balance.

VERTIGO AND THE ENVIRONMENT

Since orientation and balance can be affected as much by environmental factors as by the physical activities undertaken in these environments, people with vertigo or reduced vestibular function are abruptly made aware of properties of the natural environment which are scarcely noticed by those without orientation or co-ordination problems. An interesting example can be found in a survey of people with Ménière's disease (Austin 1992); the respondents voiced mixed opinions concerning the impact of commonly suspected contributory factors, such as diet and stress, but were almost unanimous in their observation that humid, thundery weather, and changes in pressure such as those encountered when flying, could trigger or exacerbate their vertigo (which is thought to be due to abnormal fluid pressures within the inner ear). Certain environments place special demands upon the orientation system which people with absent or distorted vestibular function may find difficult to meet. For example, walking up or down slopes alters the normal somatosensory information for postural control (based on the angle of the ankle), necessitating greater reliance on visual and vestibular information. Similarly, walking across rough terrain requires continual rapid corrections for the perturbations to balance encountered when stumbling over small holes or mounds, and these rapid adjustments are thought to be modulated partly by vestibular reflexes (Allum and Pfaltz 1985; Allum et al. 1988). Dim light, darkness, or the absence of visual structure close enough to aid in postural control (which characterises heights or open spaces) increases dependence on the somatosensory and vestibular systems (Bles *et al.* 1980; Brandt *et al.* 1980). The difficulties caused by environmental conditions such as these can become overwhelming if more than one sensory system is simultaneously taxed, for example, when walking across compliant surfaces (thick pile carpets or springy heather) in poor lighting. In addition, reduced vestibular function may promote reliance on a postural strategy of swaying from the hips rather than the ankles, which minimises the need to detect and control head movement. This strategy may be advantageous in terms of providing a steady gaze and visual reference for orientation (since vestibular input is needed to maintain a stable head and eye position during perturbations to head position), but for mechanical reasons makes it difficult to balance on support surfaces that are narrow, slippery, or moving (Dichgans and Diener 1989; Nashner *et al.* 1988).

Man-made environments can pose even greater problems, in so far as they extend the range of perceptually unusual situations that may be encountered. Many of these situations can cause imbalance or motion sickness even in healthy people who have not habituated to them; for example, most forms of passive transport result in peculiar combinations of visual, vestibular and somatosensory information that could never be produced by any normal human movement. However, the poor co-ordination associated with balance system disorders can greatly enhance sensitivity to alterations in the usual patterning or availability of information for orientation, rendering the individual both more vulnerable to travel sickness, and also susceptible to a much wider variety of perceptually confusing circumstances. One of the most common results of the enhanced sensitivity to environmentally induced disorientation described above is a phenomenon that can be termed 'visual vertigo', which is analysed in detail below.

Visual vertigo

The kinds of situations which typically elicit feelings of disorientation include: standing on a bridge with moving water or traffic below; travelling through a winding tunnel with lights flashing by to each side; traversing heights or large open spaces; observing scrolling visual displays (e.g. looking through a microfiche or computer list); walking between the long shelves of a supermarket aisle; looking at flickering lights or striped surfaces – to name but a few. These situations are characterised principally by somewhat confusing, impoverished or ambiguous visual information concerning self-motion, and an apparent discrepancy between the visual and other sources of information for orientation; hence the use of the descriptor 'visual vertigo'. For example, vestibular signals indicating head movement are usually accompanied by movement of the visual field sweeping across the line of sight (see Chapter 1). However, when observing a scrolling screen or looking down on flowing water the movement of the visual field is not accompanied by any vestibular signal. Conversely, when travelling in a lift there is no visual information to indicate movement (as the lift cannot be seen to move), but the vestibular system registers the abrupt accelerations as the lift ascends or descends. People subject to visual vertigo are often particularly disoriented in circumstances which evoke vigorous vestibular signals in combination with the unusual pattern of visual information, for example, riding rapidly over hills and bumps or around sharp bends in a car. Visual vertigo can be an isolated complaint, but many (though not all) people with diagnosed vestibular disorders also report heightened sensitivity to perceptually ambiguous situations.

Vertigo occurring in visually unusual or complex environments is a phenomenon which is poorly understood by patients, clinicians and researchers alike. It may therefore also be underreported; clinicians are less likely to elicit descriptions of these symptoms since they do not carry any clear diagnostic implications, while patients are often in-completely aware that their disorientation is provoked by specific situa-tions, or may be cautious about speculating about the aetiology of their dizziness during a medical history. My personal impression, since developing an interest in 'visual vertigo' and discussing it with a wide range of people, is that it may be more common than is generally appreciated, both within the population of patients suffering from vertigo and among people who have never been diagnosed as having any specific balance system deficiency. However, because of the apparently mysterious nature of this form of disorientation, the initial onset of visual vertigo is generally experienced as sudden, strange, inexplicable, and sometimes frightening:

> I went to the garden centre one day, and there was this huge stack of plastic pots, and somebody had tapped them and they were swaying like this [gestures from side to side] – the next thing I knew, I was swaying almost along with the pots!

> I had to come down a long, long escalator, [suddenly] I felt dreadful – I felt I was going to go tumbling all down the stairs and there was nothing I could do about it. I clung on to the escalator for dear life. Once I got to the bottom I continued my journey and tried to forget

all about it. But what it did to me was it instilled an awful fear of having to face one of those long escalators and I have a son who lives in London with a baby and there have been times when I should have been able to go – I haven't told anybody, but I feel so frightened of these escalators that it puts me off even going to London.

The woman who provided the preceding account had never visited her son in the ten years since this incident, and had not explained to her son or husband why this was. However, in all other respects her attitude to the problem was very positive and practical; she deliberately practised riding on small escalators in shops, and taught herself to reduce her disorientation by fixating on the side of the escalator. She had also found that symptoms could be caused by traffic going by as she crossed a road, heights, and being surrounded by tall buildings, and she had experienced some minor spontaneous attacks of vertigo (and a gradual onset of hearing loss and tinnitus). Her method of coping with the dizziness was to sit down or grab for support, breathe deeply, and wait for it to subside. She wasn't sure exactly what caused her symptoms, as their appearance was quite unpredictable, and had never sought medical advice since she was 'basically a believer in trying to live with what you've got – I fight it myself if I can'.

The account given by this woman does not suggest a neurotic or weak person, and yet the fear which accompanies visual vertigo is often attributed to personality characteristics. Brandt (1991) has described a common syndrome which he classifies as 'phobic postural vertigo', which combines vertigo provoked by environments with relatively complex or unusual combinations of multisensory information for orientation (such as driving, or walking over bridges, through large shops, or down stairs) with symptoms of panic, anxiety and hyperventilation. Brandt suggests that the syndrome is caused by a transient misperception of orientation information caused by anxious introspection in people with an obsessive or hysterical personality, but presents only speculative and anecdotal evidence in support of his hypothesis.

In contrast, several psychiatrists and psychologists have proposed that fear and disorientation caused specifically by disorienting environments is likely to have an organic neurophysiological basis (Blythe and McGlown 1982; Jacob et al. 1989; Marks 1981). In order to discriminate general anxieties and phobias from discomfort experienced only in situations characterised by unusual or ambiguous perceptual conditions, Jacob et al. (1989) employed a questionnaire to measure what they call 'space and motion phobia'. The questionnaire asked about responses to activities or situations potentially disorienting to those with balance difficulties, and for each of these included a 'validity' item consisting of a corresponding situation less likely to be disorienting. For example, the effects of a moving elevator were compared with those of the less disorienting (but equally claustrophobic) environment of a stationary elevator. Jacob and colleagues examined patients with a diagnosis of panic disorder and symptoms of imbalance during or between attacks, or of giddiness between attacks. They found that the items likely to disturb people with orientation system deficiencies were endorsed much more often by these 'panic' patients than were the validity items. They also found that the incidence of some (usually minor) abnormality on vestibular testing among the panic patients was twice that of a control group of healthy subjects (Jacob 1988). Levinson (1989) also reports a high incidence of abnormal neuro-otological test results in patients referred to a psychiatric department because of fears or 'phobias' relating to heights, open spaces, darkness, crowds, and various forms of travel and motion.

A similar debate has been conducted regarding disorientation experienced chiefly when driving. The label 'motorist's vestibular disorientation syndrome' was used by Page and Gresty (1985) to describe a rather specific constellation of symptoms associated with driving in particular environments: i.e. an illusory perception of vehicle motion occurring mainly when descending or turning, especially when the availability of visual information outside the vehicle is limited, such as in flat, open country, or when going over the brow of a hill. These authors found minor abnormalities on neuro-otological testing in patients with this form of disorientation, and suggested that it might be due to a failure to compensate fully for a sensory dysfunction. In contrast, Baloh and Honrubia (1990) attribute the same symptoms to 'psychophysiologic dizziness' associated with psychiatric illness, owing to the ambiguity of neuro-otological findings and the observation that many such patients develop a profound fear of driving. However, although wariness of difficult orientation tasks and environments is often characterised as phobia, such anxieties may be quite rational, as is evident from the following account given by a person initially diagnosed by her doctor as agoraphobic, but later found to have Ménière's disease:

> No way could I keep my balance or feel confident just to walk along the path, you know, that was the awful bit. I was sort of wobbling around all over the place, my balance was awful, and I was sort of walking along by the fence or something like that, keeping on to the

fence. I can remember going out and sort of fixing my eyes on the lamppost and going from one lamppost to the other lamppost . . . I tripped, and because my balance wasn't good I fell, and I fell on my head and I had eleven stitches over my eye, and broken glasses, and damaged my arm, and all sorts of things.

A plausible explanation for the phenomenon of visual vertigo is that individuals with distorted or reduced vestibular function may become dependent upon the visual system for postural stabilisation (Black and Nashner 1984b; Keshner and Allum 1986). This renders them vulnerable in situations with sparse or ambiguous visual or somatosensory information, or when rapid correction for momentary imbalance is required. The perceptual strategy of relying on visual information for orientation in preference to vestibular is logical during and shortly after vestibular dysfunction, when the signals from the vestibular system are indeed unreliable; the strategy only becomes maladaptive if adhered to after changes in vestibular function have ceased, and in situations where visual information is unavailable or unhelpful. Evidence in support of this explanation was provided by a longitudinal study of patients undergoing surgery to destroy unilateral vestibular function; immediately after the operation, half of these people developed an abnormal sensitivity to visual information, which disappeared in every case over a period of three months, as compensation for the vestibular imbalance caused by the operation progressed (Black et al. 1989).

Descriptions of visual vertigo generally highlight the apparently vague, inexplicable and unpredictable nature of the phenomenon, which seems to be a major cause of its association with anxiety in the minds of clinicians and patients alike:

Coming on the station, I walked through the station and it really bothered me – the height, the people moving and something about it, maybe the light. Light affects me, when I walk quickly out of one light to another – it seems to affect me, whether it is my mind or not I don't know . . . going through different lights, if I am prepared – I go through two tunnels on the [motorway] and that affects me, but I get prepared. I know what is going to come out at the other end and it doesn't bother me now, but it did at first because I was driving along and I wasn't really thinking about it.

An understanding of the perceptual causes of visual vertigo could help sufferers to predict and cope with their disorientation, which might therefore appear less strange and capricious. Many people do eventually develop a partial awareness of the triggers for their vertigo, as shown by the following explanation for the sensations experienced when riding in a chair lift:

> Funnily enough, I am all right going up, I can do things going up; I can go up an escalator and perhaps go up a slope, it is just the coming down part. I have to work round not being able to go down an escalator. I have had to choose a route that I can get home without having to go down an escalator, which is inconvenient, very inconvenient. So we get in [the chair lift] and we are going up and it stops halfway and it is hundreds of feet up, and [her companion] says 'Look, isn't it lovely' and I can't look – he tells me what it is like which is fine. When we got to the top he asked me how I felt and I said 'That was not bad . . . Tell you what, I will ride down.' Well, we got in, and it was fine until it started to swing out, and the actual swinging out movement . . . I tensed up obviously, my hands were sweating like crazy, and I tolerated it, but I was glad to get off.

This woman accurately notes that it was the combination of downward travel, the added vestibular stimulus of 'swinging out', and perhaps her anxiety, that induced her symptoms, but was (understandably) unable to identify the precise perceptual reason why descending should be more disorienting than ascending. In fact, perceptual explanations can be provided for most of the phenomena described by people with visual vertigo. Since disorientation can be caused by the absence of stable visual structures close enough to be used to monitor orientation and control balance, descending is most problematic, as the stable visual structures of the ground immediately above fill the visual field when ascending a slope, but when descending one looks further into the distance below. Looking at the sides of an escalator when descending is therefore not immediately helpful for controlling balance, since they are moving relative to the step on which one is balancing (although fixating on the hand-rail which moves with the step could possibly be effective). Looking at the striped treads of the escalator is also inherently disorienting, as the stripes induce an ambiguous perception of depth (Cohn and Lasley 1990). However, in the longer term, *practising* looking at the moving sides of the escalator while balancing on the step may be an excellent way of learning to reduce dependence upon visual information for orientation (see Chapter 6).

From the preceding example, it is clear that tactics which minimise disorientation at the time it is experienced are not always truly adaptive; as in the case of movement-provoked vertigo, the short-term strategies used to prevent disorientation can actually retard long-term compensation. Together with avoidance of disorienting environments, one of the most common strategies adopted is fixation on stable objects:

> I try, when I'm at home, to keep my vision fixed on something solid. You don't watch butterflies or stuff like that 'cause if you watch it flitting around it makes you go all queasy – you have to try and keep yourself fixed on something stable all the time.

Indeed, Hood (1970) has noted that people with long-standing vertigo and anxiety often become adept at using fixation to suppress the eye movements induced by vestibular stimulation. However, it is this very reliance upon a stable visual environment that renders these individuals vulnerable to visual vertigo in situations where fixation is impossible or inappropriate.

Psychosocial aspects of a changed relationship with the environment

Since vertigo and imbalance arise partly as a result of the interaction between the characteristics of the environment and the particular perceptual-motor difficulties and strategies of the individual, environments can differ greatly in terms of the hazards they present and the handicap they impose. Many people with vertigo are troubled principally by its effects on their ability to cope with a specific set of circumstances which, although discrete and relatively uncommon, are nevertheless central to their way of life. Often these circumstances are occupational; a sailor must have good balance, a construction worker must be safe at heights, a physical education teacher must be able to move freely, those offering mobile services must be able to drive, factory workers must cope with potentially dangerous machinery, and computer operators must tolerate scrolling and flickering visual field motion. Sometimes the home situation may be a source of problems; for example, living in a tower block brings difficulties with lifts or stairs to prominence, while living in a remote rural area may make driving a virtual necessity. Hence, the disability and handicap experienced by individuals with vertigo is determined crucially by their local and occupational environments; a bank manager living in a quiet town might be able to adapt with relative ease to a degree of vertigo which would completely disrupt the life of a travelling salesperson based in London.

Changes in the relationship with the environment at the perceptual-motor level also entail fundamental phenomenological changes in the way in which the environment is perceived. In her autobiographical analysis of the impact of multiple sclerosis, Toombs (1992: 54–5) comments:

> The meaning afforded by sensory-motor experience is a direct response to the world and is prior to any act of reflection or conceptualization . . . Locations and perceptions are immediately apprehended in relation to my body placement without being made explicit. Beneath objective space is a primitive spatiality of the body.

She notes that illness can transform spatial relations: locations formerly perceived as 'near' become unattainably distant, while disability may even undermine the upright posture which distinguishes every mature adult capable of 'standing on his/her own two feet'. The unsettling nature of these alterations in the relationship to the environment are vividly conveyed by the following accounts of the effects of vertigo:

> We've got an en-suite loo, and I'm lying in the bed feeling I want to be sick and go to the loo, and I mean I couldn't even walk from here to there to be sick in the loo, I had to go on all fours to be able to just make it to that door – that was to me the horrendous side of it.

> You feel that the world is no longer stable and that it's – I would imagine that it's a similar sort of feeling as if you've been through a very serious earthquake.

> You're not sure where your feet are going, and if you come to a bit of pavement that's just a little bit sloping or something, it tips your balance that much and you just go over. I found I was a bit unsteady walking, and then when I fell into the bushes on the way to work I realised things weren't – you know. I got stuck in a bush, and I didn't know what to do, I was going further down 'cause they were sort of flimsy bushes and they were just breaking off (there's still a hole up there, even now), so I had to get on to the floor and then sort of crawl, crawl out backwards and stand up again.

Hence, in the same way that vertigo can result simultaneously in disability and changes in the physical self-image of sufferers (detailed in the first section of this chapter), disorientation and imbalance may also lead to profound changes in the actual and perceived nature and possibilities of the physical environment. Van den Berg (1987) illustrates this phenomenon in normal life with the example of fatigue. Tiredness not only makes distances *seem* longer and steps steeper to the exhausted individual; these distances and heights are *actually* more difficult to scale than when well rested, and may eventually even become impassable. Similarly, to the individual with vertigo an invitation to embark on a cross-country walk at dusk no longer promises simply a pleasant recreation, but also threatens stumbling and effort owing to the difficulty of maintaining balance on uneven ground with diminishing visual information, while a trip to the city offers not only the attractions of shopping, but also the hazards of travel, crowds, busy streets, escalators and flashing lights, all of which may provoke or exacerbate disorientation.

SUMMARY

The purpose of this chapter was primarily to analyse the perceptual-motor basis of disorientation and imbalance, and to describe the physical and environmental factors affecting the experience of disorientation. However, a subsidiary aim was to begin to demonstrate the multidimensional and interactive nature of the factors contributing to vertigo. Hence, the first section explained how restriction of physical inactivity is not solely determined by physical incapacity, but is partly due to expectations and interpretations concerning the significance and likely consequences of symptoms. Moreover, such 'anticipatory disability' may actually induce physical incapacity, by retarding compensation and inducing secondary symptoms. The following sections confirmed and elaborated the reciprocal links between activity, environment and disorientation, showing how perceptual-motor activities and skills, in the context of previous and current exposure to specific environments, can influence both vulnerability and adaptation to disorientation. Finally, reactions to potentially disorienting properties of the environment and the effect of disorientation on the relationship to the environment were considered.

The interacting components of the experience of disorientation and vertigo are not confined to physical activities and environments. Indeed, even from the analysis of just these aspects of disorientation presented above, it is clear that the physical parameters of the experience of vertigo are intimately linked to psychosocial elements of the experience: the apparently inexplicable disorientation induced by visually complex man-made environments promotes anxiety and phobia, while the physical and social context of modern society offers limited opportunities for perceptual relearning; disability may give an impression of lack of spontaneity and premature ageing, while fear of the consequences of physical movement can retard compensation. The following chapter consequently explores in greater detail the way in which cognitive and emotional processes – thoughts, perceptions and feelings – influence and are shaped by the problem of dizziness and imbalance.

Chapter 4

Thoughts and emotions

The close link between vertigo and anxiety has been recognised for many years; indeed, one of the earliest explanations for agoraphobia explicitly attributed the aetiology of the syndrome to vestibular dysfunction (Woakes 1896). Numerous cross-sectional studies have documented an association between recurrent vertigo and emotional disturbance, whether assessed by questionnaire, case-study or by diagnostic interview (e.g. Eagger *et al.* 1992; Hinchcliffe 1967; Lilienfeld *et al.* 1989; McKenna *et al.* 1991). Explanations for the association between vertigo and distress have tended to be dichotomised into two principal hypothesised mechanisms: somatopsychic or psychosomatic. From the somatopsychic perspective, anxiety and distress are regarded as the consequence of vertigo and disability, whereas the psychosomatic argument is that psychological factors – whether long-standing personality traits or current stresses – may be partly responsible for dizziness or complaints of dizziness. Since most previous research into vertigo and anxiety has been couched in the language of the psychosomatic versus somatopsychic debate, the first section of this chapter reviews the evidence in support of each perspective, combining a critical review of the research literature with the introspective insights of sufferers. This overview exposes the methodological shortcomings of previous research, which preclude any definite conclusion concerning putative causal links between anxiety and dizziness, and highlights the need for an approach which examines *how* anxiety and vertigo might be related.

The following two sections are consequently devoted to a detailed exploration of the mechanisms which might mediate the association between dizziness and psychological state. Pre-conscious forms of anxiety are considered first, in an analysis of the possible role of conditioned fear responses and heightened psychophysiological arousal. The third section then identifies the features of vertiginous symptoms that are likely to induce anxiety; in particular, the unpredictability of symptoms, uncertainty as to their significance and how best to cope with them, and concern about the possible social consequences of an attack of vertigo.

The final section approaches the association between stress and dizziness from a new perspective, examining the possibility that the task of overcoming disorientation may demand significant mental effort, resulting in a reduction in the information-processing capacity available for competing mental activities. This could account for the fatigue and poor concentration frequently described by people with vertigo, and might also explain why dizziness sometimes appears to be exacerbated by mental stress.

THE PSYCHOSOMATIC VERSUS SOMATOPSYCHIC DEBATE

Personality and vertigo

No clinician would deny that psychological problems can be caused by vertigo (somatopsychic causation). Pratt and McKenzie (1958) recorded twelve instances of patients who developed various forms of psychological disturbance apparently as a direct consequence of a vestibular dysfunction; panic attacks, fear of travelling and depression were the most common sequelae. In ten of the twelve patients treatment and explanation of their medical condition resulted in recovery or significant improvement. Three of these patients had received extensive psychiatric treatment before the organic basis for their anxieties was recognised, and Pratt and McKenzie note that if no objective evidence of vestibular dysfunction is present when patients are examined there is a risk that the dizzy patient may simply be regarded as anxious or neurotic. Indeed, Marks (1981) coined the term 'space phobia' to describe the condition of a subgroup of patients referred for treatment for agoraphobia who, on investigation, had balance system disorders initially dismissed as insufficient to explain their anxiety; he suggested that in these patients an organic instability might be the primary cause of their fear of open spaces and falling. There are obvious similarities between this 'space phobia' and the development of what Levy and O'Leary (1947) have called 'street neurosis', a fear of going out (especially alone) which can develop after recurrent attacks of vertigo, which many of those interviewed in my studies readily admitted to:

I lose my confidence about going out – it's the thought of going out and one of the attacks coming on. You tend not to do things in case something happens . . . you tend to wait until somebody can go [out] with you.

I got to the stage where I was scared to do anything; I was frightened to go out, because I didn't know how I was going to be, I was frightened to get up and do anything.

Although the somatopsychic effects of vertigo are widely acknowledged, in the research literature more attention and energy appear to have been devoted to exploring the psychosomatic perspective, in particular, the idea that personality traits and/or stress may predispose the individual either to vertigo itself, or to complain of vertigo. The hypothesis that certain personality types are particularly vulnerable to vertigo has been most extensively investigated in the context of Ménière's disease. The evidence in support of a supposed psychosomatic contribution to the disorder consists mainly of studies showing that groups of Ménière's patients have higher average scores on scales measuring such personality traits as neuroticism, anxiety and hypochondriasis than do control groups, either composed of healthy individuals or of patients with other complaints assumed to be of equivalent severity (for a review, see Jakes 1987). However, Crary and Wexler (1977) point out in an excellent critique of the early literature that most of these studies failed to employ an adequate control group, and that those that did properly control for the symptom of vertigo found no significant intergroup differences.

In an exceptionally large and thorough study of the association between vertigo and anxiety, Crary and Wexler themselves assessed personality traits and symptoms of vertigo in patients with Ménière's disease, a non-vertiginous control group of patients with hearing loss, and a vertiginous control group comprising people whose vertigo was caused by conditions not suspected of psychosomatic causation, such as vertigo related to middle ear disorders, postural provocation, cervical disorder or acoustic neuroma. A battery of scales was administered, including the Minnesota Multiphasic Personality Inventory (MMPI) and various measures of anxiety, stress, and self-esteem. Compared to the non-vertiginous controls, *both* vertiginous groups had elevated mean scores on some scales, particularly the depression, hypochondriasis and hysteria scales of the MMPI. However, there were no systematic significant differences between the scores of the Ménière's disease group and those of patients with vertigo due to other medical conditions. Crary and

Wexler concluded that the psychological distress noted in Ménière's disease patients was also a concomitant of a wide variety of forms of vertigo, and was therefore probably of somatopsychic origin.

A fundamental problem besetting attempts to resolve the debate as to the putative role of psychosomatic factors in Ménière's disease has centred on the difficulty of selecting an appropriate control group for comparison with Ménière's patients. To allow for the possibility that the somatopsychic effects of vertigo may influence scores on scales measuring psychological status, the psychological profile of people with Ménière's disease has been compared with that of people with other disorders, or with different forms of vertigo. For example, Stephens (1975) found that Ménière's patients had significantly higher scores on the 'obsessionality' and 'depression' scales of Crown and Crisp's Middlesex Hospital Questionnaire than did patients with 'idiopathic peripheral vertigo'. Unfortunately, the precise nature of the vertigo experienced by this latter group was not described. In contrast, when Brightwell and Abramson (1975) compared a group of Ménière's patients with vertiginous controls they found no inter-group differences in scores on the Eysenck Personality Inventory or the Cornell Medical Index. This was despite the finding that, as in Crary and Wexler's study, the vertigo in the Ménière's group appeared more severe and handicapping than in the non-Ménière's group according to a range of self-rating measures (frequency of attacks, time since last major attack, day's work missed, etc.). In order completely to cancel out the effects of somatopsychic processes, controls should be matched on all potentially relevant factors, including the severity and frequency of vertigo, associated symptoms such as hearing loss, and the overall duration of a history of dizziness. In practice, this degree of matching is almost impossible to achieve, since Ménière's disease is normally diagnosed largely on the basis of symptomatology, and therefore precise matching by symptoms tends to yield a control group which may itself contain many individuals with suspected Ménière's disorder (Hinchcliffe 1983).

Some studies comparing groups of people with vertigo of mixed aetiology with non-vertiginous controls have also failed to uncover any substantial differences on scales assessing personality or general emotional disturbance (Hallam and Hinchcliffe 1991; Skovronsky et al. 1981). Where reliable relationships between vertigo and abnormal scale scores are established, these are usually based on a correlation between reported dizziness and somatic and phobic anxiety (Hallam and Stephens 1985; Rigatelli et al. 1984; Skovronsky et al. 1981). However, interpretation of these correlations is complicated by the risk of 'criterion confusion' created by the item content of the scales used to assess somatic and phobic anxiety. Measures of somatic anxiety almost invariably include items assessing symptoms such as dizziness and nausea, which even the least anxious vertiginous patients are bound to endorse, while scales assessing 'phobia' are not designed to take into account the possibility that the respondent may have quite rational grounds for avoiding certain situations and activities (see previous chapter). Consequently, an artifactual relationship between vertigo and somatic anxiety and phobia may be found when people with vertigo but little anxiety nevertheless truthfully report that they often feel disorientated, avoid heights and travel as much as possible, and experience attacks of cold sweating. Similarly, people with vertigo due to vestibular disorder may well report unexpected, terrifying attacks which include symptoms such as dizziness or unsteadiness, nausea, trembling, and sweating, yet these very same symptoms meet the strict psychiatric (DSM-III-R) criteria for a diagnosis of panic disorder *if* 'it cannot be established that an organic factor initiated and maintained the disturbance'. The proviso that evidence of organic dysfunction is needed to exclude a diagnosis of panic disorder therefore assigns a critical differential diagnostic significance to tests of the balance system, but these can provide only an insensitive and unreliable appraisal of balance system function (see Chapters 1 and 2).

The hypotheses and arguments concerning the nature of the association between vertigo and anxiety that are rehearsed in the research literature are also deliberated by people suffering from vertigo. The strong psychosomatic position, that complaints of vertigo are signs of underlying psychological disorder, are usually anxiously refuted (see Chapter 2), and many sufferers espouse a clearly somatopsychic perspective:

> You almost experience, as I say, a personality change. You become very insular and very introspective . . . it was everything, total underconfidence, you just don't feel like doing anything, you just want to curl up and crawl away and forget about it.

However, others are sympathetic to the idea that personality might affect the impact of vertigo:

> I think if you were the timorous type or the agoraphobic type it would be very easy to get yourself in a state where you wouldn't do things, in case.

This interactionist position, whereby psychological factors are portrayed as influencing responses to vertigo of organic origin, offers a possible explanation for the relatively high incidence of previous psychiatric problems observed in vestibular patients referred to specialist neuro-otological clinics (Eagger *et al.* 1992; McKenna *et al.* 1991); whereas the vertigo of these patients may be quite unrelated to psychological factors, the people who are eventually referred for expert help may be predominantly those who are more liable to become anxious or who have poor coping skills. There is also some evidence that the complaints of mild dizziness or imbalance which can be elicited from people who have not sought medical assistance on account of vertigo may be influenced by personality or emotional factors (Hallam and Stephens 1985). This was demonstrated in an ingenious study (Stephens *et al.* 1991) in which a community sample were asked whether they had any problems with hearing or dizziness. There was a tendency for those who admitted to dizziness also to complain of hearing difficulties, yet objective assessments indicated that their hearing was no worse than that of people who denied any hearing or balance problems. It therefore seems logical to infer that their complaints of dizziness may also have been exaggerated.

Some investigators have attempted to establish whether personality contributes to the more severe vertigo seen in hospital out-patients by asking them about their psychiatric history prior to the onset of the vertigo (Eagger *et al.* 1992). The difficulty with this approach is that persistent vertigo may result in a 'retrospective reporting bias', whereby patients who are currently distressed because of vertigo may selectively remember episodes of stress and anxiety preceding the onset of vertigo, and erroneously perceive and describe themselves as having always been abnormally anxious. The way in which anxiety and depression can influence memory and self-image has been well documented in psychiatric patients (e.g. Beck and Clark 1991; Hallam 1976). Moreover, Coker *et al.* (1989) have obtained evidence indicating that current symptomatology influences dizzy patients' self-reports of their personality characteristics. They administered the Minnesota Multiphasic Personality Inventory to people with Ménière's disease, and noted that only those who had experienced symptoms within the previous three months had markedly elevated scores; the scores of Ménière's patients who were in remission were not significantly higher than a control group of non-vertiginous medical patients.

Stress and vertigo

The hypothesis that stress, rather than personality, may trigger attacks of vertigo is also widely entertained, and is often transmitted to patients (see Chapter 1). After conscientious introspection, many people with vertigo nevertheless feel obliged to reject this suggestion:

> I know I don't get it with worry, because when I am worried about anything I don't get any attacks. When I know I am terribly worried about anything, I don't actually get an attack at that time.

However, it is interesting to note the variety of responses to a question-naire survey of people with Ménière's disease (Austin 1992), in which respondents were explicitly requested to list 'Stress factors that make your condition worse (emotional/physical)'. Despite the strong implicit suggestion conveyed by this heading that stress was likely to be a contributory factor, several people nevertheless denied any link between their vertigo and stress, writing:

> Stress factors do not appear to make condition worse – when obvious stress happens – no vertigo!

> Possibly an additional factor – but I cannot honestly say I have noticed any special correlation beyond over-exertion, or just plain end of day fatigue.

> (Austin 1992: Appendix 10)

On the other hand, many people wholeheartedly agreed with the pro-position that stress was an aggravating factor, commenting that:

> Stressful job makes it [vertigo] worse.

> Stress or being over anxious main factor. Tiredness, overdoing things.

> Stress is my biggest problem. Sudden emotional shocks, i.e. friends or relatives dying. If I work a lot of overtime then I run the risk of bad attacks.

> Stress, I'm sure, does make some difference. If I worry a lot over something (unfortunately I usually do) I definitely don't think it helps. Getting tired isn't good either especially for my tinnitus.

Stress is a problematic concept, which can been defined solely in terms of physical or psychological threats or changes caused by external events (Rahe 1988; Selye 1950), but may also be considered to embrace the individual's reactions to environmental conditions (Lazarus *et al.* 1985). From their replies, it is clear that several different definitions of 'stress' may have been employed by respondents; some people emphasise environment and life events (occupational demands, traumatic negative events) whereas others note the contribution of personality and appraisal (e.g. tendency to worry). In addition, the reported stresses very often confounded emotion, exertion and fatigue, and therefore the possible independent effects on vertigo of physiological arousal and excessive demands on information-processing capacity (see following sections) cannot be distinguished.

The answers of some respondents suggest that awareness of the psychosomatic hypothesis may have led them to search for confirmation of a causal link between anxiety and dizziness, despite the lack of any obvious association:

> I feel stress can be a factor in triggering off an attack but probably comes in a subtle and delayed way, not necessarily immediately.

> Anxiety sometimes seems to make the condition worse, but this is far from predictable.

The possibility that knowledge of the hypothesised contribution of stress to vertigo may motivate deliberate efforts to discover evidence for psychosomatic causation complicates the interpretation of research into this topic, since this increases the likelihood that occasions of coincident vertigo and stress will be selectively attended to, remembered and reported. Research into the association between stress and vertigo is consequently susceptible to problems of biased reporting similar to those which have plagued studies of personality and vertigo. In order to avoid the problems of inappropriate control groups and retrospective reporting bias, a strong test of the hypothesis that stress causes, exacerbates or triggers vertigo therefore ideally requires a prospective longitudinal design.

The study by Crary and Wexler (1977) is the only investigation which has examined prospectively whether direct links between specific occurrences of stress and vertigo can be observed. Participants in this study who suffered from Ménière's disease were asked to keep a daily record of the incidence of stressful events and vertigo. Over three-quarters of the days with vertigo occurred in the absence of *any* reported stress, either during, or for five days preceding or following the vertigo. The incidence of stress in the absence of vertigo is difficult to gauge from the reported data. However, the proportion of days in which stress neither preceded nor followed vertigo seems remarkably low, indicating that the relative incidence of reported vertigo (compared with reported stress) may have been so high as to preclude sufficient isolation of the effects of episodes of vertigo and stress. The incidence of stressful events was slightly lower before than on, or after, days with vertigo;

unfortunately, it is not possible to tell whether stress occurring on the same day as vertigo preceded or resulted from the dizziness. Finally, within-subject comparisons revealed no difference in state (i.e. current) anxiety scores at the start or end of a month free from vertigo or a month in which vertigo occurred, although the occurrence of vertigo did significantly affect patients' perceptions of whether their illness was improving (recorded at the end of the month).

In conclusion, Crary and Wexler's wide-ranging and conscientious study did not provide any clear indication that stress or anxiety can trigger vertigo. Nevertheless, the hypothesis of an immediate causal role for stress cannot be absolutely refuted on the basis of these results, partly because of the limitations of this single study, detailed above, and also because failure to prove the experimental hypothesis cannot be taken as confirmation of the null hypothesis (that stress does not cause vertigo). In addition, a basic shortcoming of the majority of investigations into the possible contribution of psychological factors to vertigo is that they have simply attempted to document an association, rather than attempting to understand the processes and mechanisms which might mediate this relationship. The following sections therefore consider in more detail the complex ways in which vertigo, anxiety and stress may be interrelated.

IMMEDIATE FEARS, ASSOCIATIONS AND AROUSAL

A sense of confusion, fear and incapacity is a recurrent theme in almost all descriptions of an acute attack of vertigo; indeed, fear appears to be an immediate, unthinking component of the experience itself. This may be partly because vertigo entails not only extremely unpleasant sensations of nausea and malaise, but also loss of control over the body, a form of helplessness which seems to be particularly strongly related to the development of anxiety and depression (Mineka and Kelly 1989). Certainly, in their explanations for the dread induced by vertigo, many people identify the incapacity and powerlessness associated with severe malaise as the most aversive aspect of an attack:

> I worry more about the attacks coming on than not being able to hear, yes, because that doesn't hurt me – the sickness and the illness does. I can accept being deaf, and the noises in my head, but what is really bad is feeling so dreadfully ill and helpless.

> I was terribly frightened, because I was completely out of control, there was nothing I could do about it. I just hate being sick, and I'm

very, very rarely sick; I think, apart from the Ménière's, only perhaps once in my life, so it's frightening.

It's just the anticipation of that, that's worst, and knowing that there's nothing you can do about it, that you weren't going to feel very well at the end of it – not life-threatening, but you were going to feel very, very ill and you were going to be two or three days, certainly twenty-four hours that you were just incapacitated.

Vertigo disrupts the relationship between self and environment at the most fundamental level, and thereby undermines the very basis for meaningful experience; as Giorgi puts it, 'all experiences are double-grounded – on the side of the world and on the side of the body . . . the crux of the matter is that the body [in active relation to the world] is the taken-for-granted ground of every experience we have' (1977: 96). Rigatelli and co-workers point out that the 'precariousness of the self' induced by vertigo is such that vertigo has been employed frequently in literature and philosophy as a symbol and metaphor for existential anxiety and confusion (Rigatelli *et al.* 1984). Indeed, some people find the experience so terrifying that they feel their very existence is threatened:

In a really bad attack I don't really know if I'm going to come round from it, you feel, you know, 'Am I going to die?' – you feel that bad.

When these attacks do come on they are frightening because you do feel so absolutely horrible . . . I felt ever so bad about it 'cause I was just stopped by the side of the road, and I was just sick, I couldn't help it – it did bother me. It's a bit frightening when you're on your own and you feel like this, and you don't really know what to – well, you can't do anything. I thought I was going to die, well, I at one time thought it was going to get me in the end, but I don't think it's that sort of thing, and anyway we've all got to go some time – but it's not a pleasant thought, is it?

Pre-conscious and conditioned fear

Of course, many illnesses evoke fear, whether of discomfort, physical decay and disability, or death. However, such fears are generally the result of conscious, and often rational and realistic, appraisals concerning the possible future consequences of disease. In the case of acute vertigo, terror often seems to be an almost automatic, instantaneous reaction, occurring at what some psychologists would consider to be a pre-attentive or pre-conscious stage of information-processing (Lazarus

1991; Leventhal and Mosbach 1983) which mediates the formation of basic associations between events and emotions (as in classical conditioning). An interesting, although hitherto untested, possibility is that disorientation may be one of the elemental dangers to which humans have been attuned by evolution, in the same way that we appear to be particularly prone to detect and fear spiders and snakes (Öhman and Soares 1993).

It is also conceivable that personality factors might operate at this stage to influence reactions to disorientation, since there is evidence to suggest that pre-conscious awareness and processing of possible threats is enhanced in anxious or emotionally reactive people and animals (Eysenck 1991; Marks 1987). Brandt has suggested that a predisposition to anxiety may play a significant role in the development of visual vertigo, claiming that:

> Neurotic acrophobia results when physiological [i.e. environmentally provoked] height vertigo induces a conditioned phobic reaction which is characterised by a dissociation between the objective and subjective risk of falling . . . Phobic vertigo syndromes require both neurotic structure of personality as well as the eliciting stimulus situation, which is often uncomfortable even for healthy subjects. Consequently, impairment of postural balance, due to ataxia or the deficiency of any one of the stabilising sensory systems, may facilitate the induction of acrophobia or agoraphobia in predisposed subjects.
>
> (Brandt 1984: 452)

Thus, while Brandt recognises that people with orientation system deficiencies are more vulnerable to 'physiological visual vertigo' than are healthy people, he nevertheless insists that only those with a predisposition to conditioned fear reactions will subsequently develop a dread of disorienting situations. In his review of the relationship between panic disorder and the vestibular system, Jacob (1988) also takes the view that vulnerability to disorientation due to vestibular dysfunction is not a sufficient cause for fear and avoidance of eliciting situations, although he terms secondary fear of disorienting situations a '*pseudo*agoraphobia', and is more tentative in attributing it to 'some other variable, perhaps personality factors related to anxiety proneness [which] constitute a moderating influence on the somatopsychic effects of vestibular dysfunction' (Jacob 1988: 366). Nevertheless, there are many situational factors attached to visual vertigo which could provide an equally adequate explanation of the development of fear and avoidance of disorienting situations without recourse to supposedly neurotic personality traits (see following section).

Jacob also outlines a (purely hypothetical) model of conditioned responding which might partly explain visual vertigo in people who have had one or more acute attacks of vertigo of vestibular origin at some time. He proposes that the intense fear associated with disorientation caused by a vestibular disorder may become conditioned to more mildly disorienting situations. In other words, having experienced the terror of a true vestibular attack, the individual may find that the first signs of disorientation – even if now due to disorienting *environmental* conditions – are enough to automatically trigger severe anxiety. Of course, this pre-conscious activation of anxiety may also be reinforced by conscious fears of the onset of an acute attack if the individual is unaware of the environmental cause of their disorientation (see Chapter 3).

A further possibility is that some form of classical conditioning of the autonomic symptoms associated with disorientation may also occur. Interestingly, Morrow *et al.* (1991) have found that the incidence of (conditioned) vomiting in anticipation of chemotherapy is related to motion sickness susceptibility, and suggest that a 'preparedness for associative learning' may mediate both. The possibility of some form of conditioned responding, akin to learned taste aversion, seems particularly plausible in view of the hypothesised evolutionary function of vertigo as a response to ingestion of poisonous substances (Triesman 1977). This might partly explain why motion sickness is often wrongly attributed by sufferers to the effects of fumes from food, petrol or tobacco (Lawther and Griffin 1988). However, Challis and Stam (1992) have questioned the evidence for an association between motion sickness susceptibility and conditioned nausea, claiming instead that awareness of somatic symptoms of anxiety arousal is one of the foremost psychological predictors of anticipatory nausea and vomiting. In a recent longitudinal study of hospital out-patients diagnosed as suffering from balance system dysfunction, the reported frequency and severity of somatic anxiety-related symptoms was also shown to predict reported change in vertigo severity and handicap (Yardley 1994a; Yardley *et al.* 1994a). The way in which somatic anxiety and autonomic arousal may influence reactions to vertigo therefore deserves more detailed consideration.

Psychophysiological arousal

Physical symptoms characteristic of somatic anxiety include sweating, muscle tension, heart pounding or racing, disorientation or dizziness, trembling, and, in extreme cases, urge to urinate or defecate and nausea (e.g. Crown and Crisp 1979; Derogatis *et al.* 1974; Schwartz *et al.* 1978). Since *all* of these (except urge to urinate) have also been described as part of the symptomatology of vertigo or motion sickness (Graybiel 1969; Morrison 1984; O'Connor *et al.* 1988), it is very difficult to determine, either in general or in the case of a particular individual, to what extent the autonomic symptoms associated with vertigo are directly triggered by disorientation or reflect the existential anxiety that also forms an integral part of the syndrome. However, statistical techniques can be employed to identify clusters of interrelated symptoms, and to determine how these symptom clusters relate to anxiety and handicap. Analysis of the responses of patients with diagnosed vestibular disorders to a questionnaire (the Vertigo Symptom Scale) assessing a wide variety of symptoms commonly associated with vertigo revealed four clusters of symptoms (Yardley *et al.* 1992b). Unsurprisingly, one of these symptom clusters related to prolonged vertigo, together with postural instability, nausea and vomiting, while a second cluster described more mild, transient sensations of disorientation; these symptom clusters were not correlated with any measure of anxiety. However, two additional, anxiety-related, clusters of symptoms could be distinguished, the first comprising symptoms which are consistent with anxiety arousal, and possibly hyperventilation (e.g. heart pounding, sweating, feeling faint or short of breath). The second cluster contained a wide diversity of symptoms (e.g. back pain, chest pain, difficulty concentrating), many of which were derived from pre-existing scales measuring 'somatisation'; high scores on the sub-scale created from these items would therefore suggest overreporting due to excessive attention to physical status, emotional distress, or general concern about health. A follow-up of the patients who originally completed the Vertigo Symptom Scale showed that the self-report measures of autonomic symptoms and somatisation were the best longitudinal predictors of subjective well-being and change in handicap (Yardley 1994b; Yardley *et al.* 1994a). These symptoms predicted change in vertigo severity over the seven-month period better than any of the other variables assessed, including age, gender, diagnostic classification, vertigo severity or duration, audiovestibular test results, or medication use.

There are several ways in which somatic anxiety and autonomic symptoms could contribute to perceived vertigo severity and handicap. High scores on the self-report measures of symptom frequency might simply indicate an excessive awareness and fear of physical symptoms. It has been suggested that the tendency to focus upon oneself is inevitably associated with distress and handicap, either because anxious self-monitoring of one's physical status is itself a sign of underlying psychological difficulties, or because constant self-evaluation draws attention to somatic and psychological states which could be interpreted negatively, and which might otherwise have been overlooked (Bass 1990; Schwarzer and Wicklund 1991). Hence, sensitivity to vertigo could be enhanced by an internal focus of attention, or by a predisposition to evaluate sensations and events as potentially threatening, or to detect and monitor perceived sources of threat (e.g. Ingram 1990; Miller 1990; Watson and Pennebaker 1989). However, although most theories of the relationship between anxiety and preoccupation with physical symptoms characterise an inward attentional focus as an anxiety-related personality trait, several of the accounts given by people with vertigo in this book indicate that they felt that their illness made them unusually introspective (see pp. 68, 70, 112).

An interactive model of the relationship between anxiety and symptom perception has been proposed by Clark (1986) to explain the development of panic; he suggests that negative perceptions of the physiological signs of arousal can themselves give rise to heightened anxiety, leading to an escalating cycle of symptoms and fear of what they might signify. For example, temporary increases in heart rate which are actually within the normal range may be interpreted as an indication of severe illness or imminent incapacitation, resulting in further anxiety and increases in heart rate (Pauli et al. 1991). In addition, many people who experience panic attacks also develop agoraphobia, as they learn to avoid situations in which they fear they might panic. In the case of vertiginous patients, autonomic symptoms may originally form part of the syndrome of spontaneous acute vertigo, but might thereafter become part of a panic reaction to the milder disorientation provoked by movement, disorienting situations, or perhaps fatigue and stress.

Alternatively, or additionally, the high somatic anxiety and autonomic symptom scores might reflect genuine physiological arousal, or even hyperventilation (overbreathing). Arousal and hyperventilation may directly enhance disorientation via the numerous reciprocal connections between the vestibular system, cerebellum and autonomic brain-stem structures (Jacob et al. forthcoming). Some authors have suggested that arousal may inhibit central habituation and suppression of disorienting vestibular signals, or disrupt central integration of information for orientation, although the evidence is not conclusive (Beyts 1987; Jacob 1988). Certainly, the gain of the vestibulo-ocular reflex is enhanced in mentally alert subjects and markedly depressed by drowsiness (Möller et al. 1990). The effects of anxiety arousal are less well established, although Jacob *et al.* (1989) noted an abnormally high gain of the vestibulo-ocular reflex in a number of patients diagnosed as having panic disorder, and anecdotal clinical experience also suggests that anxiety may result in a very vigorous response to caloric testing without fixation, or enhanced suppression of the vestibulo-ocular reflex with fixation (e.g. Hood 1984). Central functioning may be even more severely affected if the arousal results in hyperventilation, which itself causes disorientation and confusion (Drachman and Hart 1972; Theunissen *et al.* 1986).

Preliminary evidence that reported somatic anxiety symptoms may be related to genuine physiological changes is provided by a study of people complaining of vertigo provoked by head movements, which found that elevated somatisation scores and reported autonomic symptoms were correlated with objective measurements of increases in respiration rate following head movement (Yardley *et al.* forthcoming). Once again, a vicious cycle could develop whereby autonomic symptoms initially triggered by vestibular dysfunction result in anxiety and further physiological arousal, which then augments the vertigo. Some support for this model of the relationship between autonomic symptoms and vertigo is provided by the finding that perceived change in vertigo severity was related not only to initial levels of autonomic symptoms, but also to increases in autonomic symptomatology over a period of several months (Yardley *et al.* 1994a).

BELIEFS AND COPING APPRAISALS

The preceding section was concerned principally with the way in which pre-conscious reactions to disorientation may affect the experience of vertigo, but it is important to remember that conscious beliefs and appraisals can also influence responses to vertigo, both directly and through their relationship with pre-conscious fears and arousal and with voluntary activity. Leventhal (e.g. Leventhal and Nerenz 1985) has suggested that the relevant dimensions of beliefs about illness comprise conceptions of the identity and cause of the disorder, and expectations concerning the future development and consequences of the illness. Two principal ways in which beliefs and expectancies relating to vertigo may contribute to anxiety are considered below. First, the anxiety-inducing consequences of uncertainty about the occurrence and meaning of symptoms are considered, while the second subsection describes the apprehension caused by anticipation of losing control and uncertainty as to how to cope with dizziness.

Uncertainty and unpredictability

The way in which uncertainty about diagnosis may contribute to the anxiety surrounding vertigo was discussed in Chapter 2. There is also ample evidence that uncertainty about what Leventhal terms the 'time-line' of vertigo can lead to persistent apprehension. Because of the unpredictability of attacks, some people with vertigo never feel entirely secure:

> [the confidence] has disappeared because it was always at the back of your mind, whether you were in the high street, wherever you were, that any time I bend down or turn around quickly I was – I'd just bend down to pick up a bucket and I was on the floor with an attack, and I can't say I ever got used to them, even though I had them for such a long time.

> The trouble is, you never know when it's going to come on. When I go anywhere I always think 'Well, I just hope it won't' but in the back of my mind . . . [awareness of the possibility] of it happening anywhere, 'cause it can do, but then you see if I just walk up the end of the road it could happen.

In addition, doubt about the longer-term prognosis can make it difficult to plan for the near and distant future:

> It does frighten me because not knowing would it be all for the rest of my life or will it go away? I think it has affected the way I think about the future a lot, not knowing what lies ahead. Every night I go to bed and I wonder 'Will it be better in the morning or will it be worse in the morning?' and that is every night.

> It's just the sort of feeling of 'When's it going to end?', you know, is it going to be all right or am I going to be like this for the rest of my life?

> I think that to have vertigo as well as deafness was quite a frightening prospect, to feel that perhaps my life was going to be inhibited by this, the outcome was unknown, which is – with anything would be – disconcerting.

In this respect, the uncertainty surrounding the probable course of the illness may make it more difficult to adjust and adapt to vertigo than to equally disabling but more inexorable, and therefore predictable, chronic conditions. Moreover, anxiety about the uncertain prognosis may be augmented by nagging doubts regarding the possibility that the symptoms are caused by serious disease:

A little knowledge is worrying, and you wonder what it is, whether it's a growth – but that's in moments of stupidity.

Seen in the context of these, hardly irrational, concerns, the fear associated with disorientation is readily comprehensible. The contention, outlined in the preceding section, that 'pseudoagoraphobia' resulting from dizziness may imply an anxious personality (Jacob 1988) was prompted by the observation that military personnel exposed experimentally to disorienting conditions (such as a rotating room) generally develop motion sickness *without* phobia (e.g. Graybiel *et al.* 1965). However, it should be noted that many relevant factors differentiate the experience of experimentally induced motion sickness and vertigo in daily life. The military subjects were precisely aware of the cause of their symptoms, that these were normal (indeed, were simultaneously experienced by their comrades) and had no sinister implications for either their mental or physical health. Their disorientation was predictable, and the spatial and temporal boundaries of the provoking situation were clearly defined. In contrast, ordinary people rendered unusually susceptible to disorientation as the result of balance system disorder are often unaware of the sensory system dysfunction, or even of the immediate provoking factors, which cause their vague and disturbing symptomatology. Medical professionals may be unable to discover or confirm an organic basis for their experience, or explain or predict their symptoms. These therefore come to represent an apparently arbitrary manifestation of some mysterious ailment, whose characteristics suggest the almost equally unpleasant alternatives of either a neurological or a psychiatric disorder.

Extensive psychological research has shown that an unexplained, unpredictable experience attributed to internal origin is much more likely to cause anxiety than is a circumscribed, well-understood and ultimately controllable external set of circumstances (Miller 1979; Steptoe and Appels 1989). Hence, the effect of the additional uncertainties accompanying vertigo in daily life should be taken into account before concluding that predisposing anxiety or neurosis is a necessary precondition for the development of fear of disorienting situations in people prone to disorientation because of vestibular dysfunction. Certainly, pre-existing anxiety, or a predisposition to fear physical symptoms and loss of control (McNally 1990), is likely to exacerbate any unease caused by disorientation. However, to date there have been no prospective or longitudinal studies showing that *only* those vertiginous people with high levels of trait anxiety or neuroticism develop a fear of disorienting situations. Many people might become wary if subjected frequently, unpredictably and inexplicably to levels of disorientation which we normally choose to endure only in tightly controlled situations, such as the five minutes we volunteer to travel (well strapped in!) on a fairground ride.

Control and coping

Although analyses of reactions to perceived threat often tend to assume that the fundamental cause of anxiety is an elementary fear of physical harm (e.g. Clark 1986; Pyszczynski *et al.* 1991), most people with vertigo appear to be at least equally concerned about the social consequences of vertigo (a more detailed discussion of these is provided in the following chapter). In a study of the relationship between handicap and beliefs about the immediate consequences of vertigo, 101 people with diagnosed balance system dysfunction completed a questionnaire assessing fears commonly associated with vertigo (Yardley 1994a). Three main clusters of concerns were identified: fear of losing control; anxiety that the dizziness could be a sign of serious disease; and apprehension that the vertigo might become severe and cause vomiting. Concern about potential loss of control was much more common and more closely associated with levels of handicap than were the worries about sinister or severe illness. Moreover, detailed analysis of the fears relating to loss of control revealed that anticipated social consequences such as letting people down or acting strangely in public were strongly correlated with handicap (even after statistically controlling for levels of symptom severity and anxiety), whereas belief that the loss of control caused by dizziness might lead to physical harm (e.g. fainting, falling over) bore no relationship to handicap.

In addition to the effects on handicap and distress of beliefs about the causes and consequences of illness, both Leventhal (Leventhal and Nerenz 1985) and Lazarus (1991) stress the importance of beliefs about the availability of appropriate and effective coping strategies. The most striking characteristic of vertigo in this respect is the extent to which it often seems to sufferers to offer few obvious opportunities for constructive coping. A series of interviews, and a semi-structured questionnaire which specifically solicited descriptions of useful means of actively coping with vertigo (Yardley 1991b), produced remarkably few accounts of successful methods (apart from a few ingenious tactics detailed in Chapter 6). Both in these studies and in a questionnaire survey of people with Ménière's disease conducted by Austin (1992), the overwhelming majority of responses to questions about coping described restriction of activity, with many people also recommending medication use, and some mentioning rest, avoidance of stress, and attempts to distract oneself from symptoms, often by keeping busy. However, such coping strategies appear to constitute tentative exercises in damage limitation, rather than confident and successful means of overcoming the problem of vertigo. For example, in a questionnaire study of ways of coping with vertigo, efforts to escape the vertigo by keeping busy, fantasising, talking to others, sleeping or watching television more than usual, or consuming food, cigarettes, alcohol or tranquillisers, were all associated with *greater* reported handicap and distress (Yardley 1994b). Although the explanation for this positive correlation may well be that the more handicapped people were obliged to resort to these coping measures to a greater degree than those with mild vertigo, there was no evidence from longitudinal analyses that the use of these coping strategies had any beneficial long-term effects.

One of the principal problems faced by people when attempting to cope with vertigo is uncertainty about the relative costs and benefits of remaining active or resting. Many people find it difficult to decide which of these courses of action is appropriate, even when they have a clearly prioritised goal – to minimise the vertigo:

> I think there's two ways of trying to cope with it; trying to ignore it and doing as much as you would normally do, or failing that, just be very quiet, you know, and literally go to bed.

> If I catch it in time, it will go as long as I don't try and go at a normal pace, as long as I think 'Right, I'd better sit down this afternoon and it'll pass over' – very often, within a few hours, it will do . . . You get the really violent sort of attack, but then you can get something which is really a lot more mediocre, and that's the one you should try and work through, I think anyway – if I'm feeling a bit off balance or something like that, then it's best just to go to work and work it out of your system.

However, the dilemma as to which mode of coping is preferable may be further complicated by a perceived conflict between the incompatible goals of avoiding activity which might cause vertigo and maintaining a fulfilling life-style. Powers (1973) provides an incisive analysis of the potentially disastrous consequences of trying to pursue mutually exclusive goals. Behaviour is at first directed towards one goal, but to the extent that the desired state specified by this goal is approached, progress towards the opposing but equally desired state diminishes. For example, the individual who embarks on a policy of 'carrying on as normal' may be obliged to venture into situations perceived as incompatible with the aim of ensuring physical and social safety and competence. Conversely, the person who decides to prioritise preventive behaviour may find that, in order to avoid provoking dizziness, activity directed towards many other goals (exercising, travelling – even working) must be progressively curtailed. The consequence is heightened anxiety and an increasing motivation to redirect behaviour towards the alternative goal. Eventually, if behaviour is constantly redirected as a consequence of antagonistic intentions, the individual simply oscillates impotently between the two desired states. The sense of helplessness this engenders was eloquently conveyed by many interviewees, who described their confusion and frustration at being unable both to avoid provoking vertigo and to remain active:

> I really am low at times, and I say 'Oh, what a waste of my life, what a waste of time' 'cause I like to be doing something, you know, but I know I can't, and that's it. So when I'm low, I have to get busy. I can't let it rule my life, can I? I mustn't, I can't.

> I find that some days I sit like a stuffed dummy, and I might not get it [vertigo], but how long can you sit like that?

DISORIENTATION AND INFORMATION-PROCESSING

It was noted earlier (see first section of this chapter) that subjective descriptions of an association between stress and vertigo often confound emotional arousal with mental exertion or fatigue. Indeed, since emotionally challenging events frequently do involve urgent requirements for information-processing, such as appraisal of threat and coping potential or resolution of conflicting demands, it is conceivable that it is the cognitive load imposed by distressing events that is most relevant to the difficulties experienced by vertigo sufferers when they feel stressed. Moreover, accounts of the association between cognitive effort and disorientation suggest a possible bi-directional association; not only can demanding tasks provoke vertigo, but chronic vertigo also appears to disrupt concentration:

> Well, I'm always frightened to do anything or to get involved in anything that's going to cause you a lot of stress. The concentration, that's what seems to get, upset me, as I say, like lip-reading or driving, or anything that requires a lot of thinking.

I got up very quickly and, you know, the old rotation starts, very gently, very gently, but I also find then I have the problem of remembering properly. It doesn't last long, it's seconds, it wouldn't be a minute, but I don't know – your body wants to do one thing, and your mind isn't sort of tuned into it at the same time.

You drop things, you know, your concentration goes. I find that, say, I go to pick up the sugar-bowl, and it sort of goes everywhere, and then you have to clear that up. I don't really do anything properly, because the concentration definitely goes.

To the extent that orientation can be considered a perceptual-motor skill, and habituation a learning process (see Chapter 3), the relationship between vertigo and mental effort can be readily explained in terms of limited information-processing capacity (Kramer and Spinks 1991). According to pure models of limited capacity, any task which demands attention and central processing will limit the availability of resources for competing mental tasks. Hence, processing capacity devoted to orientation and habituation will be unavailable for alternative mental activity. Conversely, high priority cognitive challenges may draw processing resources away from the task of orientation, resulting in a resurgence of dizziness and imbalance.

The possibility that disorientation and habituation may make significant demands on processing capacity offers an alternative explanation for the chronic fatigue and difficulty in concentrating of which people with vertigo frequently complain – symptoms which are generally attributed either to the non-specific exhaustion and depression caused by illness, or to pre-existing anxiety or hypochondriasis. However, there is currently very little direct evidence in support of this explanation. Grimm et al. (1989) report that after a whiplash injury which damages the vestibular organ many people experience fatigue and that performance on a wide range of cognitive tests may be impaired, but interpretation of these performance deficits is problematic because the performance of people with whiplash injuries might also be affected by their feelings of dizziness, apathy and depression, or even by slight brain damage. Moreover, examination of the performance of healthy subjects exposed to disorienting conditions (e.g. sailors and astronauts) has failed to identify any substantial performance decrements (Hettinger et al. 1990). Nevertheless, studies of adaptation to disorienting environments suggest that disorienting conditions do tend to cause fatigue even when they do not provoke dizziness, nausea or distress (Hettinger et al. 1990).

Despite the paucity of experimental evidence for the impact of disorientation upon cognitive functioning, the specificity of the cognitive deficits of which people with vertigo complain itself suggests a perceptual-motor or neuropsychological rather than an emotional or motivational explanation. A notable feature of the descriptions given by vertigo sufferers of their concentration difficulties is the frequency with which perceptual-motor tasks are, often unconsciously, identified as the most problematic. In the preceding accounts, the perceptual tasks of lip-reading and driving were singled out as a cause of difficulties, while physical clumsiness was given as an example of the effect of vertigo. Specific problems with activities involving visual perception are recounted repeatedly in descriptions of concentration difficulties:

> There was another symptom that I had with it [vertigo] as well, a lack of concentration. I could pick that [note-book] up and read those notes there – I couldn't get to the bottom of the page without my eyes wanting to stop, they just didn't want to know, I would have to force myself. Many a time I would have to put it to one side.

> I play chess – I used to play chess – and I used to be good. I used to go to the chess club, and I packed that up because I started losing concentration and losing games a lot . . . You are trying to look at the board, and things are moving around, and you think 'No, I can't put up with that' . . . I have been trying to read, you start reading the same line six times over before you get to the next line. That is the annoying part about it, I seem to be going over the same line instead of getting further down the page.

Moreover, people with vertigo are sometimes consciously aware of the mental effort that they have to devote to orientation and co-ordination:

> I am walking along, and suddenly I find myself having to concentrate to walk, it didn't come naturally – if I let myself, I would totter a bit . . . sometimes I get up from my desk when I have been writing for a while, and I really have to think about walking to the tea machine.

> Sometimes I find that if I'm not concentrating I'm suddenly going near the road or something, nearly wobbling into windows, 'cause you know it is a conscious effort all the time when you're walking about, especially outside, to keep yourself going and not meander over the pavements and things.

At a basic perceptual level, abnormal vestibulo-ocular reflex function may interfere with the fine control of pursuit and ocular stabilising mechanisms needed for reading and other tasks requiring a very steady eye (as the description of the dancing chess-board suggests), while the 'poor concentration' to which the tendency to drop things was attributed by one interviewee might be due to incoordination associated with a momentary loss of balance. In addition, it is possible that the cognitive processing necessary to overcome disorientation may occupy channels or structures specialised for visuo-spatial processing, leading to competition for resources with other mental tasks which have a visuo-spatial element. Baddeley and co-workers have argued that certain activities make particular demands on central mechanisms involved in processing or temporarily storing visuo-spatial images (Baddeley 1986); these activities include everyday pursuits such as reading, driving, and any task requiring mental manipulation of images, such as plans, maps, or flow-charts. There is evidence that controlled, attentive eye movements, hand movements to spatial targets, and auditory spatial tracking tasks interfere selectively with visuo-spatial memory, presumably by introducing competing demands for attention or capacity (Baddeley and Lieberman 1980; Baddeley 1986; Smyth and Pendleton 1989). Maintenance of an upright posture under difficult balancing conditions has also been shown to interfere selectively with performance of visuo-spatial tasks (Kerr *et al.* 1985; Yardley *et al.* 1992a), while the disorientation induced by watching a rotating disc seems to disrupt the processing of a visual image in the same way that it affects visual perception (Corballis and McLaren 1982). It therefore seems possible that the continuous effort needed to overcome disorientation, disequilibrium and disordered vestibular reflexes places a small but constant demand upon mechanisms for processing visuo-spatial information.

SUMMARY: TOWARDS A MULTIDIMENSIONAL APPROACH TO VERTIGO

As noted in the previous chapter, detailed consideration of the psychophysiological, cognitive and behavioural mechanisms which might mediate the association between the beliefs and emotions of people with vertigo and the nature and degree of their symptomatology and handicap reveals a multitude of possible multidirectional relationships. The unpredictable and embarrassing nature of vertiginous attacks may provoke anxiety and overbreathing (somatopsychic causation), which may in turn aggravate the dizziness (psychosomatic causation). Similarly, the combination of strong autonomic reactions to disorientation and a predisposition to worry about health may result in conditioned panic reactions to symptoms which were caused initially by balance system dysfunction, while the mental activity devoted to anxiously monitoring and evaluating the dizziness may actually draw information-processing resources away from the task of achieving orientation.

In addition to the possible direct contribution to dizziness of over-arousal, hyperventilation, cognitive demands, and attention to somatic changes discussed, physical symptoms may also be affected by anxiety-motivated *behaviour*. The most obvious example is the way in which avoidance of disorienting activities or environments actually prevents adaptation to the disorientation provoked by these situations, but this is not the only means by which dizziness can be partly caused by fearful behavioural reactions. For example, people who feel anxious or personally incompetent may be more likely to adopt a strategy of depending upon drugs for symptom control, but may thereby prolong their physical difficulties (since tranquillisers and vestibular sedatives tend to retard neurophysiological compensation). Alternatively, un-conscious clenching or grinding of teeth, which is a fairly common component of the psychophysiological response to environmental events appraised as stressful, can actually result in significant vertigo, amongst other symptoms (Rubinstein and Erlandsson 1991).

Analysis of the relationship between vertigo and anxiety is further complicated by the probability that psychological and physiological predispositions and illness characteristics are likely to be bound up with social circumstances. For one person, the emotional distress associated with dizziness may be connected to suspicions that friends or family might regard his or her symptoms as signs of weakness or hypochondria. Another individual may find that the unpredictability of attacks and the mysterious inability to concentrate are a source of constant anxiety and self-doubt when trying to cope with a demanding job. In the following chapter this complex picture is therefore elaborated by consideration of the wider social context, and examination of how the attitudes of other people, and social and practical demands and opportunities, can further modify the experience of vertigo and dizziness.

Chapter 5

Attitudes, stigma and handicap

Even though the previous chapters have been primarily concerned with the medical, physical and psychological consequences of vertigo, its potentially damaging impact on social relationships has repeatedly emerged as a central concern of sufferers. The principal reason for seeking a medical opinion is often to obtain the official authentication and legitimation of illness necessary in order to relieve the personal disquiet and social difficulties caused by symptoms of dizziness (Chapter 2). Part of the distress caused by disability is related to the fear that physical incapacity may be interpreted by others as a sign of ageing, lack of spontaneity, or weakness of character (Chapter 3). Apprehension about letting other people down or acting abnormally in public is closely related to the severity of autonomic symptoms and handicap (Chapters 3 and 4). This chapter therefore undertakes a detailed analysis of the social implications of dizziness, and describes how the attitudes of others can fundamentally affect the degree and nature of the handicap associated with vertigo.

The first section of the chapter explains why sufferers perceive signs of disorientation or imbalance as intrinsically embarrassing and discreditable, and notes some of the tactics used to conceal symptoms from both friends and strangers. The social problems that vertigo can cause at work are illustrated in the second section. After describing the invaluable support which the family can provide, the third section examines the potential costs of this support to people with vertigo and to their families, and explores the sometimes awkward task of reconciling parental roles with the limitations imposed by disability. The final section depicts how the desire to circumvent anticipated social difficulties, combined with a rational endeavour to avoid provoking vertigo, can lead to the development of overly restrictive self-generated rules for behaviour, resulting in unnecessary handicap, frustration and depression.

THE SOCIAL STIGMA OF VERTIGO

> I can't stand people around me [during an attack] or anything like that. I've just got to be left alone, really. I think you just feel, you know, if you could be shut up in a little room on your own you would be all right.

This statement vividly conveys the conviction, shared by the vast majority of sufferers, that vertigo is fundamentally incompatible with any kind of social relations, and is therefore best endured alone. Some people make an exception for family members, who can provide much-needed reassurance and support:

> I don't want to see anybody, just want to be quiet – you just feel that you want somebody in your family to be with you.

> I mean, as long as my husband was there it would never worry me, as long as he was here . . . the first few months when I was feeling so badly he used to pop home during the afternoons, he used to ring several times when I was home to make sure I was all right.

Nevertheless, one individual actually commented that she was relieved that she lived alone, as it gave her an opportunity to be ill in private:

> I just would go and sort of creep indoors and I would be fine in the morning. Sometimes it can be quite nice to think I feel really awful, but I can go home, crash out – go to sleep or lie down or whatever – and nobody's particularly bothered.

Of course, to some extent this almost instinctive desire for solitude stems directly from the disorientation and malaise itself; social withdrawal is thus partly an inevitable response to the physical discomfort and incapacity that vertigo entails, just as apathy, fatigue and depression are also recognised elements of the disorientation syndrome. However, from the accounts of those with recurrent vertigo it appears that apprehension about the effect vertigo may have on relationships is the principal motivation for social withdrawal. Similarly, in the previous chapter it was noted that, in a sample of hospital out-patients with vestibular disorders, handicap was more closely associated with fear of embarrassment or social inadequacy than with any anxiety about physical illness or disability (Yardley 1994a).

The concerns of people with vertigo regarding its potential social impact can be best understood by reference to the concept of 'stigma', as defined by Goffman (1963). According to Goffman, an individual carries a stigma if he or she is unable for any reason to fulfil society's stereotypic criteria for normality; stigma may consequently arise from any deviation from expectations concerning the appearance, capabilities or behaviour considered normal for a particular social identity. If this deviation is immediately obvious (e.g. physical deformity) the person is at once 'discredited'. Failings that are less obvious or may be concealed (e.g. incontinence) render the individual 'discreditable', in the sense that his or her apparently normal social identity is vulnerable. The accommodations to their status open to discreditable people differ considerably from those available to the discredited; a discredited person must adopt a stigmatised identity, while a discreditable individual may prefer the effort and risks attached to trying to 'pass' as normal to the frank stigma of admitting the discreditable attribute.

It seems intuitively plausible that people with chronic vertigo may feel themselves to be discreditable; their dizziness may at one time or another prevent them from performing various normal social functions, yet they may be able to conceal this by attempting to overcome the dizziness. However, if the vertigo and ensuing disabilities become obvious, or indeed are freely disclosed, there is the risk of true stigmatisation and possible discrimination or humiliation. It is interesting, in this context, that Nobbs (1988) specifically mentions 'anxiety that one's credibility may be questioned' as a fear commonly expressed by people with Ménière's disease. Moreover, the terms in which sufferers express their desire to avoid public knowledge of their dizziness, repeatedly contrasting 'normal' and 'natural' conduct with the 'foolish' or 'stupid' behaviour caused by vertigo, strongly suggest that they do perceive it to be a potentially stigmatising condition:

> As long as my tablets are up to date then I know that I shan't make a fool of myself, and I haven't yet, apart from one really bad attack when I was really ill, and I was really glad that it was just dark.

> My main worry about it [vertigo] is other people seeing me, because of what they might think – it does look awful.

> You don't sort of phone up your friends and say 'Oh, I've got an attack of vertigo', you just don't think about it.

> It's not really dinner-table conversation that you go divulging all over the place.

> To be honest with you, there are not a lot of people I have told that I have this problem. I just try and get by without telling them. I do have to tell

them sometimes because of certain things I can't do. I can't go up and down a lift maybe, and I will say 'I'll take the stairs and I will see you at the bottom' . . . perhaps I am embarrassed about it, perhaps deep down I think 'What a fool. People think you can't go down an escalator.'

As the preceding statement indicates, people with vertigo may feel themselves to be discredited by their inability to carry out normal activities:

When you sort of tell somebody that you can't walk along the road they look at you as though you're stupid, because it's such a natural thing to do.

In addition, most sufferers believe that it is difficult or impossible to explain their unusual and, in a sense, 'invisible' condition to others:

I think that unless you can see that there's a broken arm or leg, people can't see that you've got a difficulty. I think that it's very hard for people to realise that you've got a problem, because you can't see anything, I mean to everybody else I looked perfectly fit.

I think people are a bit worried about illness, because, I mean they don't seem to – if they're not ill themselves – it's hard I think to visualise someone who's not feeling quite right all the time.

It's not the sort of thing you normally go around saying; 'Oh dear, I nearly fell into those bushes' or 'I nearly fell back down the steps' or 'I've fallen down the stairs' or something. [You feel] a bit strange talking about feeling dizzy and noises in your head, you know, not the normal sort of conversation. It's all right, you see, if you say you've got a terrible pain in your side, or your back aches, those normal sort of things.

These accounts demonstrate intuitive awareness of the parameters which determine how others are likely to react to deviant behaviour; in particular, the disquiet caused by departures from normality which cannot be easily accounted for by visible impairment or common ailments. Many sufferers therefore assume that, in the absence of any obvious explanation for their abnormal behaviour, strangers and acquaintances are unlikely to proffer the sympathy and assistance which people with more common or conspicuous disabilities might reasonably expect to receive:

I don't think the majority of people would rush over and give you a hand, quite honestly. I think that if you were just standing there I think people would be wondering why you were like that.

Indeed, the most commonly reported bystander reactions to a public attack of vertigo are bewilderment and distancing, which provoke a corresponding profound sense of isolation and humiliation on the part of the person with vertigo:

> I was tottering, so everybody stopped and watched me tottering, and no one came over just to hold my back and stop me falling. Everybody carried on, and nobody came up and said 'Are you all right?'

While the stigma attached to deviations from normal behaviour caused by imbalance are quite sufficient to induce social embarrassment, an added problem faced by people with a little known disability such as vertigo is the risk that people will misattribute the cause of their behaviour:

> I think that if you've made arrangements to go out and then you have to put it off because you've got an attack, it's very difficult for anyone to understand unless they've had one. They might think it's an excuse – they've never said, but you wonder if that's what they feel, 'Oh, they didn't really want to go.'

In particular, the intrinsic stigmatising quality of vertigo is greatly augmented by the perceived likelihood of the vertigo being mistaken for the much more stigmatising condition of public drunkenness or alcoholism. The accounts of many sufferers confirm that this is not an unrealistic fear:

> There's always the remark when I make a joke about it and say, 'Oh, well I can get dizzy on a glass of orange juice.' There's the feeling 'Is she sort of quietly hitting the bottle?' That does worry me, because as one that hardly drinks at all it's not a very nice handle to have stuck on you at all.

> I mean, I know that there are some people that think 'They've been in a pub all day long' . . . I mean, your balance does go just a little bit occasionally, and they, well 'You've been . . . had a tipple too many' or something like that. I mean you haven't even been – it would've been nice to have had a drink, haven't even had a sniff of one . . . I mean, I bumped into a woman one day in a shop, and I said 'Oh, I am sorry, I lost my balance', and she said 'You *will* be sorry.'

Misattribution of the cause of imbalance, as the preceding account illustrates, can transform the reactions of strangers from uncertainty and avoidance to outright condemnation or even antagonism. Sufferers are aware that symptoms of vertigo are likely to be attributed to drink if any aspect of their circumstances make such an attribution plausible; attacks occurring at a party or pub are therefore very likely to be misinterpreted:

> When you [lose your balance] other people are going to – especially if you're at a party – they're going to think you're drunk . . . it's falling over in public at a place where they've got alcohol [that is worrying], and I thought 'Well, I don't want to get that sort of reputation.'

Factors such as age, appearance, and the time of day also influence strangers' interpretations of an attack on the street. As a result, a teenager who had developed Ménière's disease (highly unusual, but not unknown at his age) found that bystanders' reactions tended to be hostile:

> Some people are horrified, they do not know what to do. If they see someone who they think has inflicted this on themselves by drinking, they're going to say 'Well, sod you now, get on with it.' I think you can get passed on the street – you'd be desperately ill and people would walk past you because they think that you were drunk. Several people when they saw me thought I'd been on the bottle – I had comments on the street if I had an attack on the street.

There are several ways in which people can react to the possibility of stigmatisation. Some are determined to overcome the stigma by correcting the ignorance about vertigo that they encounter:

> I wore a Medi-aid bracelet for a long, long time with inside literally written 'I am not drunk, I'm having a Ménière's attack.'

> I think sympathy and support is very important [during an attack]. I always say to people who think I'm drunk 'Well look, I'm sorry, but I've got a problem.' I usually tell people, for instance in an office, 'Look, I've come over all queer, there's some pills in my handbag, and just leave me alone.'

Having explained their condition, many people found that they then received generous assistance and sympathetic understanding. An additional strategy, which can help to reduce the sense of personal insecurity which potential stigmatisation can induce, is to seek the company of those whom Goffman has termed the 'wise', i.e. fellow sufferers. The support which can be provided by people who have experienced the same problems is especially valuable, not only because no shame or stigma is attached to the shared difficulties, but also because the information they provide is perceived as more accurate than that given by the uninitiated (Cohen 1992). Several people commented that they felt it was, or would have been, beneficial to discuss their condition with other people who had vertigo:

> It was nice to actually meet someone else that knew what was going on or knows a similar experience, and to actually get a little bit of understanding of it. It was interesting to meet him and chat to him, it was helpful in a way . . . It was just nice to actually chat to somebody who really understood what happens, because it is all very well describing your symptoms to someone, but unless they are actually suffering with it they don't really know what the experience is like.

> I could have been helped right from the start if I could have spoken to somebody [who was a sufferer]. If you could talk to each other you could find out from each other what was going wrong and I think you would probably help somebody.

Nevertheless, the general dislike of stigmatisation is such that the majority of people with vertigo choose to attempt to conceal their infirmity from all but a few relatives or close friends:

> I'd only tell people that it would affect – I wouldn't tell people, you know, as a rule of thumb.

> I try not to talk about it. I think it's embarrassing when people keep reminding you and they say 'Well, how are you?' and 'Is it better or worse?' and you've sort of got to explain.

This strategy results in the dilemma that an unexpected attack of vertigo might at any time undermine their 'normal' identity and necessitate informing and involving people around them. One method of coping with this problem is to present some alternative, more socially accept-able, reason for any temporary lapse in normal behaviour:

> I just say I'm not feeling very well, because it's such a long-winded thing to go into, unless it's people I know. I just simply say 'I just feel a bit sick, not feeling too well, must be sickening for something.'

Another common solution is to involve selectively just one or two relatives or close friends who can be relied upon for discreet assistance:

> I don't go away with a friend or anything like that, we always go together – L [husband] understands and knows.

> If I phone a friend and she says, 'Oh, so and so is coming as well' I say 'Well look, I'll tell you how I feel so I won't have to explain to them what is wrong with me' – I hate that.

Thing with this is that if you've got a support like a husband or a wife, whichever one of you, then it is not so difficult because you can go out with them and hold on to their arm, and it's not so bad.

Goffman describes this tactic precisely, and notes that these confidants are then expected to fulfil a number of duties, including helping the stigmatised individual to 'pass' as normal. Hence, people with vertigo can avoid exposure of their dizziness by leaning on the arm of a relative when they feel unsteady, or may rely on their confidant to make plausible excuses and take them home quickly if a sudden attack occurs in public.

Despite these partial solutions to the problem of stigmatisation, as the correlation between handicap and fear of social inadequacy would suggest, many people are so distressed by the social difficulties attendant on an attack of vertigo that they simply try to avoid situations in which they might be discredited:

I'm not going to put other people in the situation if I can where I would be a liability.

Like, when we go out for a meal, I don't want to accept to go because I never know when I'm going to be bad, and you don't want to upset other people. I've had an attack in a friend's house and they were bewildered, they didn't know what to do. But my husband said, 'Just let her lie down for a minute, she's not too bad.' But of course it puts other people off. It feels as if I'm drunk, and a couple of people have said, 'She's been drinking again' and I never touch alcohol you know. You can explain it to other people, but I think unless you've got it yourself, other people don't understand what it's like. Very, very difficult. Like, if you're walking up, you're going like that [gestures a swaying motion] and people sort of look at you, you know . . .

Naturally, avoidance of social activities and roles can have serious detrimental consequences for both the individual and for the family concerned. Moreover, when these difficulties interfere with occupational roles and demands, the consequences can be especially far-reaching. The problems associated with work that people with vertigo may encounter are considered in more detail in the following section.

OCCUPATIONAL DIFFICULTIES

For most people with vertigo, the determination to conceal the vertigo and pass as normal is even stronger in the context of work than among friends or strangers. For example, one man whose general inclination was to be open about the vertigo – 'I think that if you explain to other people the problem then they understand it' – nevertheless admitted that:

> My work – shall we say that I have to keep it [the vertigo] a secret; if I was with my bosses or the people I work with, I wouldn't say a word.

However, the daily social exposure which employment entails, and the constant necessity for movement, travel, and physical and mental activity, result in a particularly high risk of being discredited. Since few sufferers are entirely successful in disguising their difficulties at work, most are eventually obliged to cope with the consequences of disclosure. Many find that their employers and colleagues are supportive, and may even adopt the role of confidant which family members play at home:

> The girls [at work] were very good, that were under me. I'd say 'Oh, gosh, I've got a funny attack' and they'd cover, you know, and we'd sort of work it together – they were very good.

Others are less fortunate, and experience a variety of forms of stigmatisation, which may even culminate in implicit or explicit pressure to leave work:

> They [work colleagues] used to fiddle their time, they would say they were sick and have time off, but we knew between ourselves what they were doing, so when I started this [vertigo attacks] they thought I was doing it, but I wasn't doing it at all. The supervisor used to sort of wonder too, because I looked so well before and after. It wasn't pleasant, because I knew I was genuine, I did think once or twice 'Oh, blow them, I'll leave' . . . [The Welfare department at work] said to me one day – one of the senior ones – she said 'Have you thought about taking early retirement for this [vertigo's] sake?' so I said 'No, I haven't really.' So she said 'Well . . .' and she sort of had a chat to me about it and said 'Well, you think about it . . .'

> There are others [work colleagues] that, um, 'You shouldn't be working', 'You shouldn't be here', 'You shouldn't be in a position of responsibility', 'You shouldn't be driving' – well, you name it. They want to get rid of me, they want to get me out of the way because it's worrying them, it's embarrassing them. My job was threatened, they wanted to retire me early against ill health. [I felt] A young man, young family, that's it, all washed up, what am I going to do? 'I'll be OK' [I'd say], 'I can carry on work, I can carry on with my shift, there's no problem, I've had my tablets, I'll be all right' – anything to reassure everybody that I was going to be OK and that the job was going to be OK.

The response of many people, as these accounts illustrate, is to redouble their efforts to demonstrate the ability to fulfil normal roles and duties. Nevertheless, some sufferers ultimately decide that it is fruitless to endure the stress and tension of attempting to live up to the practical and social demands of their occupation. In one survey of 100 patients seen at a hospital clinic for people with vestibular disorders, half of the respondents reported occupational difficulties, and 11 per cent of the sample had changed their job or left work altogether because of the vertigo (Yardley and Putman 1992). In a second study of 127 hospital out-patients, two-thirds of those who were employed stated that the vertigo caused problems at work and 10 had been obliged to change the nature of the work they did, while among the 50 who were unemployed 13 had given up work because of vertigo (Yardley *et al.* 1992d).

A variety of factors determine whether the vertigo will be compatible with continued employment. Inability to carry out necessary tasks, such as driving or scaling heights, together with repeated unpredictable absence from work, tends to create an uneasy relationship with employers and colleagues. This can itself provide the motivation to leave, as the precariousness of the sufferer's occupational status may be a cause of persistent anxiety:

> You feel that, you know, well how long are they going to employ me on the work they give me now? I mean, somebody is going to say 'Well, we can do without him because we've got to cut down on staff, and he's the first one to go', so that's the way you feel now.

The decision of some sufferers to leave work is directly due to the stress and fatigue of ill health, but others are primarily troubled by their inability to fulfil occupational duties:

> I was upset that I thought it would be stupid to put other people in my charge, and therefore I wouldn't take the job.

> I've stopped teaching, because I think the teacher ought to be able to do what she's telling the class to do, and if I can't lie on the floor it's ridiculous, because a lot of it is done down there.

Interestingly, whereas many people with permanent and substantive disabilities choose to fight occupational stigmatisation by asserting the rights of the handicapped, most people with vertigo are acutely aware of the employer's perspective:

> I always feel that if I'm employing somebody you can't afford to employ somebody who's always being ill. How many small firms

could afford me now? They couldn't, could they? So I just feel lucky that I work for a large firm.

I was off so long they couldn't – 'cause they're only a small company and they need as many people as they can get – and I was off so long they couldn't cope without me, so they had to get somebody else. I understood, because you know they have the right to do it because, you know, they can't really let their business go because I'm feeling ill.

In the case of people with temporary and partial disabilities such as those caused by vertigo, agreement with the logic and attitudes of former colleagues may act as a protection against stigmatisation in a different way, by asserting the identification of the individual with normal society, rather than with any disabled subgroup.

Nevertheless, for those obliged to give up work because of vertigo, the combined impact of the change in social roles and the abrupt drop in income could be far-reaching, as a former van-driver explained:

I am relegated to the role of looking after the house and looking after the kid and so on. Financial problems and everything associated with being out of a job – it comes quite hard . . . I worked long hours, mostly six days a week, so there was not a lot of leisure time as such, but what time there was we did tend to enjoy, but now we are very restricted in what we can do, mainly through finance . . . We did have a problem within the marriage, but that was not so much through the lack of being able to get out and socialise but more the stress of me actually being in a position where I was not working, where I could not do an awful lot. The financial worries are big, and it just all sort of built up.

In the following section, the effects of vertigo on the family, and family reactions to the problem of vertigo, are examined further.

VERTIGO AND THE FAMILY

The vast majority of people with vertigo report that a few relatives (or occasionally close friends) constitute their principal source of support, and that their help is invaluable. Comments from both married and widowed individuals suggest that the spouse, in particular, typically plays a central role in enabling them to maintain a fairly normal lifestyle. As noted in the first section of this chapter, such 'confidants' may assist the vertigo sufferer to 'pass' for normal in public and to cope with routine activities. The first two subsections below describe the nature and costs of the support provided by close relatives, while the third subsection discusses how disclosure of infirmity and the need for assistance from children is influenced by the special nature of the relationship with dependants.

Support by confidants

The nature of the support which partners, close relatives or friends may contribute is multifarious, as illustrated by the written replies of forty people with Ménière's disease to the question 'Is your confidant able to help you feel better when you are upset? If so, how?' (Austin 1992). Simply knowing that if a sudden attack of vertigo occurs there is someone who understands the problem and who will offer discreet practical aid can be sufficient to give sufferers the confidence to continue with valued pastimes and social roles; several respondents indicated that their confidant helped 'just by being there', 'just knowing someone is there is enough'. Many people also highlighted the way in which their confidant sustained them 'by sympathising and helping me not to feel guilty if I can't do things', 'by providing support and being totally understanding', 'sympathetic and tries to keep me cheerful' (Austin 1992: Appendix 8). Others noted appreciatively that such emotional support was supplemented by tangible or instrumental support: 'practical help with chores'; 'patient and understanding and a great help when I am literally on the floor'; 'moral support and practical support, e.g. doing the household chores when I have an attack, nursing me'. Indeed, the assistance required of confidants sometimes consists of actual physical support – literally, a shoulder to lean on, or help negotiating stairs or getting home.

Research into the mental and physical health benefits of social support indicates that the family may play a particularly important role in protecting individuals against the stress of illness (Argyle 1992). Jacobs (1992) suggests that open communication and shared problem-solving within the family are important, and many of the responses to Austin's survey confirmed that one of the principal ways in which confidants could help sufferers was 'by just listening', 'by talking through problems as they arise', 'just being able to talk and get my innermost thoughts out', 'by being there, sympathetic and bracing', 'being realistic about when I need to rest and when I need to be active'. As the preceding comment suggests, one of the central functions of such communication is to facilitate the negotiation and planning of changes in roles and patterns of work-sharing which illness may necessitate

(Corbin and Strauss 1985; Jacobs 1992). In addition, discussions with confidants can provide 'appraisal support' (Schwarzer and Leppin 1992); trusted intimates may thus help sufferers to evaluate the extent of the threat they face, to identify possibilities for effective coping, or to construct positive meaning in their situation. It is interesting that many confidants use the technique of 'downward comparisons' with people perceived as having worse problems in order to encourage the sufferer, according to the descriptions of appraisal support given by Austin's respondents:

> [The confidant helps when I am upset . . .]
>
> by discussing what I can still do, and how much I have been able to achieve despite the handicap of Ménière's, and how much worse it could be;
>
> listening to me, particularly tells me there are others with more serious problems, makes me a cup of tea!
>
> by letting me rest as need be and reminding me of other people (friends, relatives etc.) in worse circumstances.

In a study of women with cancer, Taylor (1983) has observed that downward comparisons appear to be an important method of bolstering the sense of mastery over the illness and enhancing self-esteem. In addition, some family members use explicit declarations to provide what Schwarzer and Leppin (1992) have termed 'esteem support', and to ensure that chronic illness does not undermine the sufferer's sense of identity and worth:

> My husband keeps assuring me of my worth within the family as this is my biggest worry, that I am becoming a burden. He tells me I still make a valid contribution and this is very important to me.
>
> [My confidants help] by stressing that their love or friendship is not conditional upon my health, i.e. by 'allowing' me to be ill.

The costs of support

The task of providing support is not without its costs; indeed, the distress of the partners of people with chronic illness tends to be correlated with the distress of the sufferers themselves, and is often of the same magnitude (Coyne and Fiske 1992). Moreover, the burden of stigma and handicap may fall as heavily on the family as on the individual

(Anderson and Bury 1988). Jacobs (1992) notes that chronic illness poses problems of 'boundary regulation' within the family; family members may be obliged to sacrifice a significant proportion of their personal time and objectives in order to take on the additional tasks created by the disability of their relative – whether the chores of daily living (housework, shopping, even paid employment) or the work specifically generated by the illness (assistance with bathing or travel, escorting the relative to medical appointments). Jacobs also remarks that chronic illness which is characterised by unpredictability may be especially disruptive to family activities, as the following account confirms:

> Obviously, we could never plan ahead to do something, say going out for an evening, because you would never know what I was going to be like on the day. You could plan three or four days ahead, but no more than that really. You couldn't plan a month or a couple of months in advance because you couldn't – I could never guarantee that I would be fit to go anywhere.

In addition, family members may be prevented from pursuing rewarding pastimes because of the inability of their afflicted relative to accompany them. The restriction of activity and limitation of social contact caused by the illness can therefore result in a substantial change in the life-style of those close to the sufferer, which may affect both their quality of life and the social support available to them:

> It tends to upset our plans and things sometimes. We used to be very active doing things, we belonged to a rambling club and we used to go barn-dancing, and we had a good social life – and we still have, but in a different way – we had to change our pattern a bit because of it [vertigo] you see.

> It's also altered his [the husband's] life quite a bit – certain things we used to do together, go for long walks, or car – I can't go in the car very often, that makes me feel bad, it can start me off. We used to go away for weekends to Manchester, drive up to friends – all that, I just can't do any more.

To the extent that the spouse or partner shares the handicap, anxiety and sense of helplessness associated with vertigo, he or she is also likely to share the consequent feelings of frustration and discouragement:

> Well, he [the husband] feels restricted as well, plus when I get these attacks he's hopeless, he can't do anything for me, and so you can see that he's anxious and he gets a bit uptight.

While most families are able to negotiate a shared solution to these problems, the strain on relationships caused by recurrent vertigo can have serious consequences, as in the case of one young man with Ménière's disease who confessed that:

> I would think that she [his wife] found it as stressful as I did at various stages . . . I suppose it ended my – or helped end – my marriage, because there were times, well, a whole year when I was worse, so I couldn't help.

Awareness of the costs of providing support to a person with chronic illness leads some people with vertigo to conceal their difficulties to some extent even from their closest confidant:

> I try not to show too much to him [the husband], I know that it pulls him down.

> Often I don't even say to my husband that I feel like it, because I seem to always be feeling like it, you know, and I don't sort of let on, you know – it's a strain to do that.

Moreover, the spouse or confidant is not always entirely supportive. The frequent absence of positive test results or diagnoses, and the vague, unpredictable nature of the symptomatology, can raise doubts concerning the authenticity of the illness even in the minds of close relatives, as two women, who both eventually received a firm diagnosis of balance system dysfunction, discovered:

> I think he [the husband] feels with me that it is sometimes self-induced, that I get worked up about things and therefore I get it.

> My husband just dismissed it in the end because nobody had come up with an answer. It was obviously me and nothing else. I think he thought I could put it at the back of my mind and it would go away.

It is possible that such reactions constitute another instance of unintentional 'victim-blaming' (see Chapter 2) provoked by the persistent and apparently insoluble problems associated with recurrent vertigo. Harris (1992) notes that confidants sometimes withdraw their support if repeated crises result in what appear to them to be excessive demands for succour, and that rejection by the person from whom support was anticipated is the most distressing form of social support failure. She also observes that criticism by the confidant frequently takes the form of accusations of overreacting to the stressor or failing to cope appropriately. Certainly, the strain of accommodating to the demands created by vertigo occasionally results in accusations either of provoking attacks by overactivity, or conversely, of hypochondria. When these contradictory accusations are levelled at the same individual, the effect is to exacerbate the classic internal conflict experienced by people with vertigo regarding the optimum balance between rest and activity:

> You feel guilty about not being able to cook, because, you know, your husband's been out at work all day – I feel very guilty. My husband will come in and get cross with me because I've tried to do it [cook a meal], which then causes a problem . . . He's very good, he looks after me very well, as long as I don't try. He really is very, very good, he gets on with the food and things, asks me if the hoover's disturbing me. If I had an attack at the weekend when he's home, he would have to do the housework and look after me and get the food. [Then] he'd be fed up when he has to go back to work on Monday, and he might mention it in the week, 'You always seem to be bad weekends' or something.

The psychological costs of having to rely on family or friends for assistance are not confined to those who provide the help. Dependence upon others restricts the possibilities for activity in numerous small but cumulatively frustrating ways:

> You can't have a shower unless somebody's there – you have to get up very early in the morning to have a shower because the husband goes to work or you have to have it in the evening before you go to bed.

> You tend to wait until somebody can go out with you – I mean that is the main problem.

Many people with vertigo also feel a sense of inadequacy, humiliation, or guilt at being so dependent:

> I don't like being taken to the loo by my husband, I think that's – even with [him] – it is so degrading, I find it demoralising, I really do – see that would upset your sort of confidence really

> You can't restrict other people all the time, because that's what you're doing, you're saying 'Well, don't leave me on my own' or you're saying 'Please come out with me' – it's very, very difficult.

> You're relying on other people so much it hurts, because you're losing all your independence. I mean, very often, I get a bit fed up of being indoors and I think to myself 'Oh, I'll go up to my mum's' and then I think 'Oh, well I've got to ask my husband during the day to

come up with me' – not that he minds, he never complains. Or we've got to go to the hospital [for speech therapy], I've been going twice a week, sometimes three times a week, he's got to leave everything and come with me. It's always relying on somebody, and you feel, as good as people are, that you're putting on them all the time. I mean, I'd give anything occasionally to go into town, walk around, look at the shops, but you've got to keep on all the time asking people – then I go, and the bus makes me feel bad, and I regret that I went.

Reconciling parental roles with vertigo

The sense of inadequacy occasioned by disability may be particularly acute when incapacity interferes with the care of offspring. Inability to meet the customary obligations of parents or grandparents because of disability is not infrequently described as a cause of guilt or humiliation (the first of the following accounts was given by a woman unable to drive because of vertigo):

> My friends drive, and I either have to depend on them or my husband. He is really good, he takes me everywhere, but it means he has to revolve his life around my life, and now I have got children as well it is making life difficult . . . until I can drive I feel I am letting my children down in a way, because they are not doing things – my friend takes her children swimming and she just goes, she doesn't have to rely on her husband to take them there, and I think they are missing out to a certain degree.

> It does affect me in so far as I feel that my daughter-in-law has two small children, and I feel that they don't ask me to take the children like they do her mother because they're afraid of my taking them in case I have an attack, and in a way I resent that.

Particular efforts are made to try to fulfil parental roles, not only in the practical sense, but more often by concealing the stigma of vertigo when in the company of the children, at school events, weddings, or on family outings. Relationships with children seem to fall within an ambiguous category somewhere between confidants, on whom the sufferer can rely for support, and the general public, who are not generally expected to know about the problem or provide help. Goffman (1963) notes that young children are generally considered too unsafe or vulnerable to receive information about a parent's infirmity, and many people with vertigo confirm that they attempt to conceal their stigmatising condition from the children:

We hid it away from the kids for a long time – Dad was having a stomach upset or had eaten something which hadn't agreed with him.

With the grandchildren I like to stay as normal as possible, I would try not to let them see, the children. I wouldn't want them to be afraid to come to Grandma as she might fall over.

Indeed, one woman described her perceptions of her growing children's changing attitudes in terms of a sequence of progressively more sophisticated stigmatisation:

At the time I think they were quite worried that Mother kept falling over. If I ever did [have an attack in public] with them around I think they would be mortified with embarrassment, absolutely mortified, and would disown me. I think now that they're that much older they probably think that I was secretly hitting the vodka.

Even when their children reach adulthood, parents are often reluctant to relinquish this protective attitude towards them, and when information about the individual's problems is disclosed to offspring there is sometimes concern that these failings might be perceived as 'inconvenient', a 'liability', or an unwelcome imposition upon them. Accordingly, accounts of adult children's reactions to vertigo suggest that while they are generally helpful, they may show less sensitivity and comprehension than the partner. For example, one recently widowed woman described her family as 'very supportive', but in comparison with the total support from a very close husband on which she had previously relied, her request for help from her son seemed somewhat reluctant, and his response slightly clumsy:

When I had the Ménière's before [the son] was being made redundant. I was so upset at his situation that I wouldn't have dreamed of impinging on it again, but I did talk to him about it, and I make light of it really – I don't want the kids to be worried about me. That sounds very noble, but perhaps it is that I don't want them to think that I can't manage on my own – perhaps it's selfish really! . . . [when she had a severe attack while living alone] I was frightened to go up stairs on my own in case I slipped on the stairs and had to be nursed, and it seemed more sensible to get somebody to take me upstairs than to risk falling. And so I rang [the son], and he came and he let himself in, and he'd come with a friend. [The son] doesn't understand it at all – how could he? Nobody can if they haven't had experience of it, and because like most kids [laughs] – at his age! . . . he's not a kid at all really, is he? But when he meets something he can't understand he makes a joke of it, it's embarrassment really, so he was saying, 'You've been at the bottle' – of course, I don't drink so he knew he wasn't going to upset me . . . and I sort of played along with it really and I said to him, 'Will you take me upstairs?'

Another woman described her difficulty in persuading her daughter, first, to accept the reality of the disability, and then to countenance measures which might reveal her mother's stigmatising infirmity:

I'm not tying them to me, we've got to each live our own lives and 'cause I didn't want to be a burden on them . . . like my daughter, she didn't have any patience with me at all, but then she realised that – now she realises as I was there for ten months, how I've had to work hard and struggle, help myself, and she realises that I did have a problem . . . She won't let me take my trolley out [for support], but I said, 'Well look, I'm going to have to hold on to your arm to cross the road, if I feel a bit wobbly then I'll have to hang on to your arm' . . . she sort of agreed to that.

In summary, a very few close relatives or friends typically provide people with recurrent vertigo with a variety of forms of invaluable support. Indeed, given the extent to which sufferers usually depend on close relatives to help them maintain a normal identity and cope with routine activity, it seems likely that the availability of such support will influence the degree of handicap arising from vertigo, although to date there has been no research on this specific topic. Nevertheless, dependence upon others can have significant costs for both confidant and sufferer, and may place some strain upon their relationship. The next section provides an overview of the relationship between attitudes, behaviour and handicap, showing how beliefs about the social and physical consequences of vertigo modify behaviour, and how behavioural responses can in turn influence the physical, social and emotional consequences of vertigo.

SELF-GENERATED RULES AND HANDICAP

The preceding sections of this chapter have illustrated how the belief that vertigo and its consequences are socially unacceptable is widespread; people with vertigo view it as a stigmatising condition, the effects of which are unlikely to be understood by others, and may indeed be misinterpreted as drunkenness or hypochondria. As a result, the preferred way of coping with vertigo is to attempt to 'pass' as normal, often with the aid of a spouse or other close confidant. The potential consequences of this strategy are threefold: first, increased levels of dependence and therefore tension in family relationships; second, a constant fear of public exposure, which can lead, finally, to a voluntary withdrawal from the social situations in which the subject feels vulnerable. In addition to concern about seeming odd, foolish, or even drunk, people prone to vertigo are often apprehensive that they may embarrass or annoy others by proving unable to keep commitments or to perform normal roles (dancing, travelling, walking at a normal pace). Some people are deeply disturbed at the prospect that at any time they might suddenly be disabled, with the concomitant embarrassment that would ensue; as one interviewee put it, 'You can't ever be confident that something's going to work out right.' A fear of being discredited therefore frequently provides the motivation for deliberately restricting social contacts and activities, as in the case of other potentially stigmatising conditions characterised by fluctuating symptoms, such as early multiple sclerosis (Robinson 1988) and epilepsy (Scambler 1989). It is interesting, in this respect, that a young man with Ménière's disease specifically mentioned that someone with epilepsy had helped him to learn to cope with his condition:

> It was, in fact, a young epileptic that I had in the unit who sort of showed me the way, and said if I was worried about having an attack I'd never get out of bed. I've got to get on with life, I've got to do it, and if it happens, it happens, so tough luck if it happens.

Another motive for retiring from a variety of social and occupational activities originates from the desire to avoid provoking vertigo (see Chapters 3 and 4), whether by exertion, travel, stress, physical or mental activity, or exposure to disorienting environments. The restrictions on life-style following from both these coping strategies tend to be formulated as self-generated rules governing behaviour, based on beliefs concerning the available courses of action and their potential consequences (Zettle and Hayes 1982). Such rules may prove truly adaptive, if they derive from an accurate appraisal of the contingencies present in their environment, and thus serve to help the individual to cope successfully with the dizziness. However, self-generated rules are sometimes based on erroneous beliefs, or are overgeneralised across situations and over time. Where inappropriate rules are based on untested or untestable beliefs they may impose maladaptive limitations and constraints upon an individual's behaviour, and a vicious cycle of self-inflicted distress can aggravate the reaction to the original problem. For example, if vertiginous attacks are correctly judged as causing specific difficulties at work this might either motivate a constructive reorganisation of working practices to cope with these problems, or alternatively might lead to the formulation of a general rule that vertigo rendered the individual unfit for work, with consequential premature and unwanted retirement.

There is ample evidence that in response to vertigo, sufferers often do formulate general rules for behaviour based on their beliefs about the probable consequences of activity (Yardley *et al.* 1992c), as in the following instance of avoidance of a pleasurable social and physical activity, given by a woman with Ménière's disease:

> I used to enjoy perhaps going to a dance, but again, there's no way I can be spun around on a dance floor now. I'm worried that if I am spun round, I'm going to, it's going to happen again, it might just bring it on. So I think 'No, I'll do what I know I'm able to, and the rest of it, well . . .'

Unfortunately, people who experience unpleasant, and apparently unpredictable, symptoms tend to apply these rules over a wider range of situations and longer time-scale than may be strictly necessary in order to avoid dizziness and social exposure. Such blanket prohibition of activity is a logical strategy for coping with vertigo which is perceived to be unpredictable, but the avoidance behaviour limits opportunities for testing or extending the boundaries of possible action, and may thus perpetuate a vicious circle of diminished self-confidence (Bandura 1982; Scheier and Carver 1988). Moreover, these self-generated rules, intended to help the individual manage his or her dizziness, can themselves become a cause of depression in so far as they exert rigid and unwanted constraints upon behaviour, often far more extensive than the direct effects of vertigo itself. The result may be an apparently insoluble dilemma, in which people are torn between the fear of provoking vertigo or being socially discredited and the desire to escape a depressingly constrictive life-style.

Powers (1973) suggests that the only escape from the dilemma of conflicting intentions is to reorganise one's value hierarchy and define new goals. Unfortunately, the consequences of such a reorganisation are not always entirely positive. A relatively common response to the psychosocial problems posed by illness is to adopt the role of an invalid. This solution gives the individual a new identity and a less ambitious set of goals, and thereby minimises the risk of failure. Such behaviour can have agreeable consequences, such as receiving attention and sympathy, or being absolved from unpleasant or stressful duties. However, the costs often include relinquishing the prospect of fulfilling many normal roles, accepting the stigma attached to this departure from normal behaviour, and putting strain on social or family relationships.

Another way in which multiple goals may be pursued is through the hierarchical 'nesting' of sub-goals (Scheier and Carver 1988). For example, the higher-order goal of maintaining an idealised self-image is translated into principles (e.g. 'be independent'), which, when confronted with a range of possibilities, motivate the selection of a particular course of action (e.g. concealing an attack of vertigo rather than asking for help). This is, in turn, executed via a variety of subordinate acts (finding something to lean on, making up socially acceptable explanations for unusual behaviour, etc.). Scheier and Carver suggest that while behaviour is directed towards a sub-goal this goal temporarily becomes *functionally* superordinate. The difficulty is that, in the process of dealing with immediate problems, it is easy to lose sight of higher-order goals. An individual may be concerned on a daily basis with avoiding provoking vertigo, or being exposed in public while dizzy, and may seldom reflect on whether his or her behaviour is detrimental to the pursuit of higher-order goals and principles, such as maintenance of an independent, fulfilling life-style and a positive self-image. As a result, day-to-day behaviour may not be consistent with the course of action that a rational cost-benefit analysis of the problems caused by vertigo might suggest. Examination of the ways in which people with vertigo attempt to regulate the impact of their condition on others reveals a clear contradiction between sufferers' expressed resolution to carry on as normal and to avoid informing or involving others, and their evident need to confide in and rely on people for practical help. This contradiction does not result from a distinction between self-reliant and dependent individuals; the same people frequently state a desire to cope alone, but also give numerous examples of receiving or soliciting assistance. There is also a clear contradiction between many individuals' expressed determination to carry on as normal and the various restrictions on activity that they are actually forced to adopt.

In some cases, this predicament may result in a condition of 'learned helplessness' which is believed by some psychologists to be virtually synonymous with depression; if the individual considers that the vertigo has aversive consequences over which he or she has absolutely no control, and if these consequences appear to be extensive and long-lasting, then depression is likely to ensue (Abramson *et al.* 1978;

Mineka and Kelly 1989). People with vertigo perceive themselves to be helpless in the sense that they are incapable of competently performing many of the social, occupational and familial roles they have previously occupied. They may be physically incapacitated at times, they are unable to engage in a variety of valued pursuits, and their dependence on others has increased. Feelings of anxiety, failure and helplessness may also result from the apparently insoluble conflict between the wish to remain active and independent and the need to limit activity and seek assistance. Moreover, a sense of isolation may be fostered by the withdrawal from social networks, as well as the belief that others are incapable of understanding their situation.

Although somatopsychic processes have been emphasised above (partly in order to highlight the fact that the association between vertigo and distress can be adequately explained without recourse to hypothetical personality disorders), it is likely that predisposing personality traits will influence the degree of handicap and distress caused by vertigo. Pre-existing levels of anxiety are likely to enhance the development of fear of vertigo and stigma, while feelings of personal incompetence may hasten withdrawal from social activities. Similarly, those with low self-esteem may be prone to underestimate their ability to cope with the vertigo, while pessimists are more likely than optimists to conclude that their problems are intractable and overwhelming. However, while self-imposed limitations on activity may reflect a failure to perceive or generate coping strategies or a pre-existing tendency to adopt a helpless, dependent role, they may equally well represent an active attempt to control the situation which then becomes maladaptively overgeneralised. Moreover, the links between personality and handicap may be bi-directional, as many people with vertigo describe personality changes which they directly attribute to the vertigo and its consequences:

> I used to be very outgoing, I worked all my life as a computer operator, I used to go out a lot, to pubs, with my husband, theatres, dancing. All that, it's out of the question now.

> I was a very outgoing person, and I have become, largely because of this [vertigo], very introverted. When you're afraid there's a risk that you might fall over it's not easy to go into a room of people you don't know. Whereas at one time I'd have breezed in and been the life and soul of the party, I couldn't possibly do that now.

The experience of vertigo can thus be seen as the product of many interacting dimensions, which all too often combine to create a vicious cycle of escalating handicap and distress. In order to reduce the risk of provoking unpleasant and frightening symptoms, and to avoid the social embarrassment and stigma they might cause, many people with balance system disorders deliberately restrict their physical activity, travel and social commitments. However, the resulting loss of valued roles, supportive social contacts and rewarding pastimes may fuel the feelings of anxiety and helplessness initially caused by physical illness. In addition, avoidance of vigorous movement and demanding perceptual environments may prolong the duration of the vertigo by retarding sensorimotor adaptation. Nevertheless, despite this gloomy depiction of the potential for disability and depression, ultimately most people with vertigo learn to adapt to disorientation and to reverse the cycle of handicap. The final chapter describes how it is possible to adjust to and overcome the problems caused by vertigo, either with or without professional help.

Chapter 6

Coping with vertigo

The purpose of this chapter is to examine how each aversive aspect of the experience of vertigo can be ameliorated, and how the vicious cycle of escalating anxiety and handicap can be reversed. Many people with vertigo either do not seek medical help or, even if they do see a doctor, draw chiefly on their own resources in order to cope with vertigo. The accounts of those with long experience of living with vertigo therefore provide an invaluable source of information about what adjustment to vertigo may involve, ranging from practical tips on how to manage attacks to hard-earned insights into how to overcome or cope with fear and disability. However, most people with significant recurrent vertigo express a desire for professional help; ideally a cure, but at least some form of advice or rehabilitation. Much of this chapter is therefore devoted to a critical evaluation of existing and potential therapies.

The fluctuating, ill-defined, and multifaceted character of the problems experienced by people with vertigo makes treatment evaluation particularly difficult. The measurement of recovery or improvement poses serious problems which have not yet received sufficient attention. Because of the ability of the balance system rapidly to compensate for vestibular dysfunction, a person who is experiencing frequent attacks of acute vertigo may be free from signs of disorder on the actual day of examination. The traditional tests of balance system function are therefore unable accurately to monitor the severity of current symptomatology. Consequently, assessment of improvement has hitherto been based almost entirely on rather crude therapist ratings which do not discriminate between the different elements of the experience of vertigo and may be affected by the expectancies of the therapist. Evaluation of therapy outcome is further complicated by high rates of (apparently) spontaneous remission and strong 'placebo' effects. These problems have also been largely ignored, and treated patients have rarely been compared with appropriate control groups. Moreover, in a multi-dimensional condition such as vertigo, unaccountable occurrences of 'spontaneous remission' and 'placebo recovery' deserve closer inspection. Spontaneous remission might actually signify the operation of unspecified processes such as beneficial changes in the attitudes, expectancies, behaviour or circumstances of the people concerned which help them to come to terms with their problems; similarly, placebo effects may result from non-specific features of therapy, such as empathy and reassurance (Stiles *et al.* 1986).

If such psychosocial factors do, indeed, have a profound impact on the experience of vertigo, then interventions specifically intended to influence these aspects of the experience might result in significant improvements in well-being. However, the range of treatments which have so far received consideration has been constrained by a narrow focus on pathophysiology. Pharmaceutical and surgical remedies have been much more extensively employed, and evaluated, than any other kind of therapy, and the possible benefits of alternative forms of rehabilitation remain largely unknown. The following sections therefore not only examine the evidence for the efficacy of conventional medical treatments, but also explore the way in which some of the difficulties experienced by people with vertigo may be reduced or averted by changes in their activities, environment (physical and social), beliefs and emotions.

The first section considers the kinds of surgery and drugs commonly used to treat vertigo, and examines the reasons for both their effectiveness and their limitations. The second section briefly reviews the burgeoning field of exercise therapy for vertigo, and outlines some of the factors influencing the choice and success of the various types of physiotherapy. In the third section, the psychological elements of the experience of dizziness are considered. Measures are suggested that might prove helpful for reducing psychophysiological arousal, promoting habituation of conditioned reactions, relieving anxiety about symptoms, and encouraging self-confidence. Finally, ways of minimising the handicap associated with dizziness and imbalance are discussed.

MEDICAL MANAGEMENT

The principal methods employed by doctors to alter or control the course of vertigo are drugs and surgery. Only a relatively brief description of the possibilities and limitations of pharmacological and surgical treatments is provided below, since a comprehensive review and evaluation of these forms of treatment is beyond the scope, and the concern, of this book.

Surgical treatments

The most radical form of surgery to eliminate vertigo is 'labyrinthectomy', the destruction of the malfunctioning vestibular organ. However, this procedure also destroys hearing in the operated ear, and 'best practice' therefore now recommends that this procedure is *only* employed when the vertigo is disabling and there is no usable hearing in the ear concerned (Paparella *et al.* 1990; Smith and Pillsbury 1988). An alternative means of eliminating signals from the disordered vestibular organ consists of cutting the vestibular nerve. This is a relatively new and delicate form of microsurgery which carries a (fairly small) risk of quite serious complications and side-effects, such as cerebro-spinal fluid leakage, facial paralysis which may last many months, permanent total hearing loss in the operated ear, or meningitis (Green *et al.* 1992; Pohl 1991; Smith and Pillsbury 1988). Nevertheless, the reported rates of success in controlling the vertigo for both these procedures are usually around 90 per cent – better than the highest placebo rates of improvement. Vertigo is occasionally caused by a 'fistula', or hole in the vestibular organ (labyrinth) resulting from either trauma or middle ear disease. In these, relatively rare, circumstances surgery may be necessary, and is generally quite effective if the tiny fistula can be identified (see Grimm *et al.* 1989; Ludman 1984).

Since labyrinthectomy and neurectomy should completely eliminate the input from the diseased organ, it is pertinent to reflect upon the possible reasons why these treatments do not achieve a 100 per cent success rate (apart from side-effects). Occasionally the surgery may fail to destroy completely the vestibular organ or nerve, necessitating re-operation. A more serious alternative reason for operative failure may be misdiagnosis; if the operated organ is not the sole, or the main, cause of dizziness, the operation is unlikely to succeed. Consequently, if the symptoms actually arise from disordered functioning of some other part of the balance system, such as the other vestibular organ, or even a non-vestibular problem, the operation will not be helpful. Worse still, if the dizziness is caused by a failure of central compensation, or by multisensory deficits, the violent vertigo initially provoked by surgically damaging the vestibular system may actually result in a long-term or permanent *exacerbation* of the problem. These possible outcomes are particularly important to consider because the published success and complication rates naturally represent the achievements of the most skilled and prestigious surgeons working in the best medical environments, and anecdotal accounts of surgical disasters in less prestigious institutions are not infrequent. One of the more common forms of misdiagnosis arises from a failure to appreciate the extent to which anxiety, beliefs and behaviour may be contributing to the patient's difficulties. When this is the case, the operation will be unable to fulfil the patient's heightened expectations, resulting in bitter disillusionment. One man, whose dizziness and anxiety were eventually alleviated by a programme of combined physiotherapy and psychological therapy, described how the failure of surgery actually intensified his fear and distress:

> I had been blaming all of my problems on to the Ménière's. Every time I didn't feel quite with it I would blame it on to Ménière's, so when I had the Ménière's operation I expected it to be better, and I got worse. The symptoms got worse: pressure in my head, pressure across here, pains in my head. My eyes were funny, I got very anxious, I thought I had real problems – hence the scan, and all the other things that I had.

Another widely used form of surgery consists of a range of procedures intended to prevent attacks of vertigo in patients with Ménière's disease, essentially by relieving the increased pressure in the fluid (endolymph) in the vestibular organ which characterises this condition. This type of surgery does not entail destruction of hearing and vestibular function – an important consideration, since about one-third of those with Ménière's disease eventually find both ears are affected. A variety of techniques are employed (most commonly, the 'endolymphatic shunt'), all of which have been reported as achieving a roughly similar success rate, averaging about 70 per cent, with fewer and less serious complications than the more destructive procedures (e.g. Paparella 1991; Raivio et al. 1989; Smith and Pillsbury 1988). In some cases, repeat operations are needed after a few years, and success rates in halting the deterioration in hearing occurring in Ménière's disease (which can be objectively measured) are significantly lower than those reported for control of vertigo.

In practice, reported rates of improvement in symptoms following shunt operations vary quite widely, ranging from 49 per cent to 90 per cent, with the better rates tending to be reported, naturally, by the surgeons who are most enthusiastic about the technique. Unfortunately, almost all of the published clinical trials have suffered from crucial methodological weaknesses, the most serious being the lack of independent, blind assessment of improvement, or absence of a suitable control group. The latter failing has resulted partly from an under-standable reluctance to withhold treatment, and partly from the assumption on the part of many clinicians that an adequate within-subject control condition is provided by the long base-line period of disabling vertigo, unalleviated by drug therapy, which generally constitutes the criterion for offering surgery. However, the course of Ménière's disease is extremely unpredictable, consisting of fluctuating clusters of attacks, which often become progressively more frequent and severe over a few years, and then tend to become milder and less frequent, eventually ceasing (Haye and Quist-Hanssen 1976; Stahle *et al.* 1989). Consequently, a certain rate of improvement may be expected on the basis of statistical probability alone. Moreover, the 'placebo' effects associated with surgery are generally ignored, even though they may constitute important aspects of the treatment. Features of undergoing surgery which might affect the experience of illness include: the recognition and sanctioning of the individual's status as truly and seriously disabled, and the consequent removal of the stigma associated with suspected hypochondria; a hitherto unparalleled level of attention, interested sympathy and explanation; communication of the belief that the ultimate form of treatment has been provided; and possibly advice or therapy to assist compensation after the operation (see, for example, the recommendations for pre-surgical counselling of the patient given by Bägger-Sjöbäck 1988). Indeed, in the only double-blind, placebo-controlled study of endolymphatic shunt surgery, the same success rate – about 70 per cent – was observed in both the active and the placebo groups, and no significant between-group differences in vertigo or hearing levels were present at a three-year follow-up (Thomsen *et al.* 1983). (However, some surgeons have argued *post hoc* that the placebo operation, which did not involve the vestibular organ itself, might nevertheless somehow have affected the physiology of the surrounding region in a relevant fashion; see Smith and Pillsbury 1988.)

Pharmacotherapy

The much larger literature on pharmacological treatment for vertigo cannot reasonably be reviewed here. Nevertheless, the limitations of drug therapy are implicit in the lack of consistent agreement as to which treatment is superior, and for which symptoms, the persisting requirement for surgery in a significant minority of patients, and the admission by most authors that drugs can offer only symptomatic therapy (Dix 1984a; Hanson 1989; Paparella 1991; Paparella *et al.* 1990; Pykkö *et al.* 1988). Diuretics and betahistine are both reputed to reduce the severity of attacks of vertigo experienced by some people with Ménière's disease, although they are probably unable to eliminate the vertigo or halt the progression of the disease (Dix 1984a; Paparella 1991; Paparella *et al.* 1990; Ruckenstein *et al.* 1991), and restriction of salt, water, alcohol, nicotine and caffeine are also often recommended. However, Brandt (1991: 48) notes 'The existence of a large number of therapies [for Ménière's disease], each supported fiercely by its advocates, usually indicates that there is no demonstrably effective therapy available.' Schmidt and Huizing (1992: 181) concluded an exhaustive and well-conducted comparative trial of betahistine with the statement that there was no evidence that it was superior to a placebo, and the comment that:

> The improvement that is reported in the majority of studies lies within the range of 60–80 per cent, regardless of type of therapy. As long as a more effective treatment has not been found, one should choose the least noxious therapy available. At present, participation in a trial seems to be the best treatment of Ménière's disease.

Although there appears to be no effective prophylactic pharmaceutical treatment for vertigo, a variety of drugs may help to alleviate the experience of acute vertigo by partially suppressing the activity within the vestibular system or by inhibiting the autonomic symptoms associated with severe disorientation, although these drugs are not generally considered suitable for long-term usage, particularly as they may retard or prevent central compensation (Pykkö *et al.* 1988). Those commonly prescribed include antihistamines and phenothiazines (e.g. cinnarizine, prochlorperazine) and tranquillisers (e.g. diazepam); anti-motion sickness drugs may also be tried (e.g. scopolamine), and haloperidol, phenobarbitone and meclizine have also been recommended (Dix 1984a; Hanson 1989; Paparella 1991). The non-specific effects of many of these drugs upon the central nervous system are frequently viewed as a useful means of simultaneously reducing the anxiety which accompanies vertigo. Indeed, the philosophy guiding pharmacological treatment of vertigo is succinctly expressed by Paparella (1991: 117):

> Medical therapy treats certain symptoms or [*sic*] the patient, thereby circumstantially improving conditions for the patient but not treating the disease per se. Since the action of most drugs has an empirical basis, it is our policy not to discourage the use of any of them if the treatment minimizes the symptoms and improves the quality of life for the patient.

In this approach to medical management, the difficult task of attempting to distinguish between 'placebo' effects, somatic or psychological effects, or, indeed, the coincidence of spontaneous remission, is largely abandoned, and a wide range of drugs may be tried in a pragmatic effort to find a treatment that appears – for whatever reason – to suit an individual patient. Moreover, because of uncertainty as to the physiological mechanisms whereby these drugs may exert beneficial effects, coupled with awareness that their benefit may often be due to central sedative or placebo effects, patients are seldom given the unambiguous information they would need in order rationally to evaluate and regulate their usage of medication.

The aim of the preceding overview of pharmacological and surgical methods of treatment for vertigo is not to deny their usefulness, but to draw attention to the limitations and uncertainties that render these forms of therapy an incomplete solution to the problems that vertigo can pose. The clinicians and authors who prescribe the medical treatments reviewed above are, of course, by no means insensible to these limitations, and themselves emphasise the need for supplementary forms of support for the patient. For example, Paparella (1991: 117) precedes his survey of medical therapies for Ménière's disease with the statement that 'Psychological support with patient education may be the most important part of medical management'. Similarly, Bägger-Sjöbäck (1988) introduces his paper on the surgical treatment of vertigo with the recommendations that, before even broaching the subject of operations, the patient should be given continuity of care with a doctor who can guarantee support in any emergency, and an opportunity must be provided for in-depth discussion of the nature of the patient's condition and how best to adapt in order to live with it. In the following sections these aspects of therapy, and other means of coping with vertigo, are given the serious, detailed consideration that they merit.

EXERCISE THERAPY

Since the 1940s a series of clinicians and authors have advocated the use of exercises to promote central compensation following a vestibular lesion (Dix 1984b). The dominant rationale is to provide a structured opportunity for recovery of multisensory and sensorimotor co-ordination over a wide range of orientations and movements (see Chapter 3). The exercises which the individual is asked to perform are intended to include those eye, head or body positions and movements which provoke vertigo (or, on the principle of limited generalisation of compensation, at least a representative sample of these provocative motions). Adaptation should thus be enhanced or accelerated by repeated experience of the conditions which are found disorienting – in the same way that, with repeated exposure, one adapts to environments which initially cause motion sickness.

Clinical trials of the efficacy of exercise programmes typically report improvement in symptoms in over 80 per cent of those participating, but with complete elimination of vertigo in less than a third (Hecker *et al.* 1974; Norré 1988; Norré and de Weerdt 1980; Shepard *et al.* 1990). (Improvement refers to a reduction in movement-provoked vertigo or residual dizziness and unsteadiness, as exercise therapy is not expected to reduce the number or severity of spontaneous episodes of acute vertigo.) Most of the trials of exercise therapy suffer from methodological shortcomings similar to those criticised in relation to evaluation of surgery. Very few have employed an adequate control condition, and 'improvement' has generally been assessed by the clinician responsible for treatment, using rather crude and limited criteria, and ignoring such considerations as therapist effects (Crits-Christoph and Mintz 1991) and the definition of clinically significant change (Jacobson and Truax 1991). For example, Norré's measure of improvement simply consists of a reduction in the proportion of nineteen test positions which elicit complaints of vertigo (ignoring real-life subjective well-being or handicap), while Shepard *et al.* (1990) evaluate pre- and post-therapy disability on the basis of the therapists' ratings on a single five-point scale.

Some of the more recent studies are beginning to remedy these shortcomings. Horak *et al.* (1992) have undertaken a comparison of vestibular exercises with medication (valium or meclizine) or general conditioning exercises. Preliminary results indicate that both assessments of postural stability and subjective ratings of symptom severity show more improvement in the vestibular exercise group than in the other two treatment conditions. Shepard *et al.* (1993) also found a higher rate of improvement among people recovering from vestibular neuritis who were given exercise therapy than among those who had an operation to section the vestibular nerve. In a preliminary comparison of relaxation therapy with vestibular exercises, Savundra *et al.* (1993) found that while both groups improved, the vestibular exercises resulted in a more significant reduction in movement and position-related vertigo, assessed by blind therapist ratings.

The varying and often incompletely specified patient selection procedures used in many of the clinical trials render it difficult to determine the overall success rate that might be expected in a heterogenous clinical population. The majority of studies explicitly exclude all but the most clear-cut and uncomplicated cases of position-related vertigo, although Shepard and colleagues report that rehabilitation helped people with a wide range of symptoms and diagnoses. More disconcertingly, only one of the studies referred to above has addressed the issue of drop-out or non-adherence rates. Savundra *et al.* (1993) note that more than a third of the patients in their study failed to complete the therapy programme. It is parsimonious to assume that the reported success rates in the remaining studies refer to only those individuals accepting and completing the rehabilitation programme. Perhaps the prestigious and highly motivated centres involved in these clinical trials were able to achieve a negligible rate of non-compliance with their recommended therapy. Nevertheless, the issues of acceptance and participation deserve close attention, if only to determine how such high credibility and completion rates are sustained, since many people are disconcerted and disappointed to be offered, instead of a miracle drug or surgical cure, a therapy which requires them actively to induce the very symptoms that they dread:

> I was sceptical at the beginning. To begin with, I didn't realise it was so simple to correct, and after having it for years I couldn't see how overnight the thing could change. Because it was so simple in the way of exercises, I couldn't imagine in my brain that that was going to fix it. To be honest, I know this sounds stupid – I mean people don't like going to hospitals – but I thought an operation or something would fix it. That was the only way I could imagine it to work . . . My husband thought I was crazy, basically, because he thought the exercises were so simple I probably didn't need to do them at all anyway.

> I went to a neurologist. He talked to me, threw me around a bit on the couch, asked me how I felt, and said, 'Go away. Try some exercises.' Which I failed at miserably, I didn't do them very well at all. I hardly did them, because I was frightened, I only did them a couple of times, because I was so frightened of getting dizzy at that time I just couldn't do it. [The doctor] said if it didn't work for me, then he would refer me to [a specialist clinic]. So I did cheat a bit, because I just couldn't face doing them. Because he didn't have time to talk to me, time to explain to me. I was still frightened, I was still worried, I needed someone to have some patience.

As the preceding account suggests, failure to complete a physical therapy programme is often not admitted to the doctor who recommended it. The consequence of such covert non-adherence is that doctors receive a poor impression of the effectiveness of exercise therapy and may refer fewer patients, or even reserve it for intractable cases. They may also unconsciously communicate their low expectations for success to those they do refer, resulting in even lower rates of completion and a reduction in the placebo improvement which most therapies for vertigo achieve.

A comprehensive evaluation of any form of rehabilitation ideally demands an empirical, fine-grained analysis of precisely how therapeutic processes may relate to particular problems and outcomes (cf. Newman and Howard 1991). Given the limitations of the empirical evidence from clinical trials, the following discussion of the relative merits of various types of exercise-based therapy for different forms and aspects of vertigo is obliged to draw upon personal clinical experience, theory and deduction. These suggest that the benefits of exercise-based therapy may have many dimensions, ranging from alterations in neuro-physiological function to promotion of confidence and a sense of control.

In certain cases, head and body movements may actually be able to affect the physiological cause of vertigo. 'Benign paroxysmal positional vertigo' (see Chapter 1) is triggered by changes in head and body orientation or by linear accelerations such as starting or stopping in a car, and is believed to be due to the accumulation of debris at certain locations within the balance organ (Schuknecht 1975). Some clinicians claim that by performing particular head movements very briskly, which should dislodge and disperse the debris, this kind of vertigo can be completely eradicated in over 90 per cent of suitable patients (Häusler and Pampurik 1989; Herdman 1990). Others have found it difficult to replicate this success rate (Parnes 1993), and debate continues as to the best technique of this kind. In particular, since the head movements concerned are those that provoke vertigo, some authors have suggested that the mechanism responsible for recovery is actually central compensation, which can be achieved by a longer, more gentle series of movements (Norré and Beckers 1987), although the very rapid recovery rates that often occur (after only a few head movements) provide evidence in support of the hypothesis of peripheral structural changes in at least some cases. In an excellent review of these forms of physiotherapy, Herdman (1990) suggests that the selection of technique should be based on a multifactorial assessment of the individual, rather than on theoretical predilections. The factors she lists as relevant include restrictions on violent movement imposed by other conditions (e.g. arthritis) or by anxiety, and the ability or willingness of the individual to pursue a protracted programme of exercises.

Relaxation techniques are also sometimes taught to people with vertigo, for a variety of reasons (Beyts 1987; Ödkvist and Ödkvist 1988). When dizziness is related to neck tension, hyperventilation, or jaw-clenching or grinding, or is provoked by stress, relaxation may directly remove a cause of vertigo. Alternatively, relaxation training (with EMG biofeedback) has been suggested as a means of increasing tolerance of the symptoms provoked by exercise-based therapy (Leduc and Decloedt 1989), in the same way that autogenic feedback training can reputedly help people to cope with disorienting motions (Cowings and Toscano 1982). Re-education of postural control, in order to eradicate postural habits which contribute to instability or muscle tension, may also help to reduce imbalance or vertigo at source. Encouragement to participate in sports or other vigorous activities also features towards the end of many therapeutic programmes, in order to reverse the general loss of fitness and mobility that often accompanies chronic vertigo, and to enhance orientation and motor skills.

Debate continues as to whether exercise programmes need to be tailored to the sensorimotor capabilities and specific difficulties of the individual concerned. Although generic exercise programmes, which include the movements that most people with vertigo find problematic, achieve good results with the majority of those who complete them (e.g. Hecker *et al.* 1974; Shepard *et al.* 1993), Norré claims that exercises are only effective in so far as they include practice with those positions and motions that the individual finds disorienting. Norré and de Weerdt (1980) found that the symptoms of patients who performed exercises which did *not* provoke vertigo remained unchanged, but after the same patients had practised performing disorienting movements their symptoms improved. This study, albeit somewhat anecdotally reported, is interesting because it included a within-subject control condition. From the start, these patients had (presumably) received the explanation of vertigo and compensation which Norré considers an indispensable precursor to therapy (Norré 1984). Moreover, performance of even non-provocative exercises should have also provided those participating in the programme with expectations of improvement and control, and a sense that the clinician was taking an active interest in their problems and believed that they could recover. Nevertheless, it was only when the provocative movements were made that improvement in symptoms of vertigo became evident, indicating that this improvement could not be attributed to the effects of reassurance and psychological support, but depended upon recovery of sensorimotor co-ordination through activity.

Shumway-Cook and Horak (1989) also advocate programmes of physiotherapy tailored to the individual's particular pattern of maladaptive sensorimotor functioning. For example, people who seem to rely excessively on visual information for orientation are asked to practise balancing in environments where the visual cues are absent, unusual or ambiguous, while those who rely mostly upon somato-sensory information practise walking on compliant or moving surfaces. Specific training in motor strategies suitable for different balancing tasks may also be useful. For example, a motor strategy commonly adopted after attacks of vertigo is to lean and sway only about the hips, and not around the axis of the ankle joint (perhaps because it is possible in this way to keep the head upright and hence avoid provoking or using vestibular signals). Since swaying from the hips exerts sheer forces between the feet and surface of support that will lead to falls on slippery or narrow surfaces, people who use this strategy exclusively need to learn how to sway from the ankle when necessary. People with complete loss of vestibular function may require special exercises designed to hasten the development of new forms of eye–head co-ordination. They can also benefit from education in recognising and coping with environ-ments in which they will inevitably find it difficult to balance; i.e. those characterised by an absence or paucity of visual and somatosensory information (Shepard et al. 1990).

In view of the situation-specific nature of the incoordination asso-ciated with vertigo (see Chapter 3), specially tailored exercise pro-grammes have high face validity on theoretical grounds. Perhaps equally importantly, individualised programmes may have high face validity for the individual concerned. Tailoring an exercise programme entails working with the individual to discover his or her particular sensorimotor weaknesses, selecting exercises that directly address these, and discussing how the exercises may be expected to affect particular forms or aspects of disorientation and disequilibrium. The process of identifying those movements or perceptual conditions that provoke vertigo provides a concrete demonstration that the programme is relevant to the person's problems, which tends to promote confidence in the therapy. Moreover, this process helps to establish a good relation-ship with the therapist: one which encourages active sharing of infor-mation and of responsibility for exploring diagnostic and rehabilitative possibilities and progress. As a result, the individual is likely to achieve a more profound, and constantly developing, comprehension of the nature of his or her problem and the possibilities, difficulties and limita-tions pertaining to adaptation, and should consequently be better able to monitor, predict and control the course of recovery. This goal is quite explicit in some tailored programmes. For example, Shepard et al.

(1990: 470) state that, in addition to promoting compensation and teaching postural control strategies, the 'major thrust' of their therapy is:

> To educate the patient in techniques for helping to manage their symptoms and functional deficits. They should understand that therapy is *not* a cure for their balance disorder, but simply a management technique ... if taught a means for dealing effectively with recurrent symptoms, the patient can re-institute the techniques independently.

The comments of one man, made after completing only a few weeks of exercise therapy, suggest that the provision of a means of dealing with vertigo is appreciated, even when a complete cure is not guaranteed:

> It has changed my outlook on the way I have been coping in the past. As to whether it has any lasting effect, I don't know at this stage, but obviously we will have to carry on and see. But overall, I think it has probably helped to a certain extent, I mean, already the exercises have been getting easier so obviously I have been compensating better – so time will tell. I mean, previously I was just sort of shuffling down and just sort of letting the world go by, until I felt I ought to do things. Obviously now, because of the theory behind it, I am going to push myself to actually try and overcome it with the use of the exercises ... I mean, obviously having a goal is important, so I think it is going to be helpful.

The possible multiple benefits of tailored therapy considered above suggest that it is impossible to equate several aspects of the therapeutic conditions when employing exercises which do not provoke vertigo as a control condition for comparison with exercises which *did* provoke vertigo. Thus, the demonstrable superiority of the provocative exercise programme may not be entirely attributable to its ability to enhance compensation; expectations, confidence and motivation may have been higher once exercises which could be seen to affect the vertigo were included in the therapy. Indeed, although this section has focused principally on adaptation in terms of recovery of sensorimotor co-ordination, repeated experience of vertigo in the safety of a therapeutic environment may itself confer additional benefits beyond an actual reduction in disorientation or disability. In particular, it provides an opportunity to explore the nature and boundaries of the experience itself, the provoking factors, and coping mechanisms. This opportunity is likely to result in a reduction in uncertainty and anxiety, and recovery of a sense of self-control. Indeed, many people explicitly mention the motivation and confidence promoted by exercise therapy as a major benefit:

It is nice to have some way forward in all this . . . I have come to accept now that there is something that I am going to have to deal with forever, but to my mind [exercise therapy] is giving me something that I can work with, whereas before all I have had is a full-stop there; 'You have got that problem – basically, tough! Go away, there is nothing we can do about it.'

Before [having therapy], I tried to block it out and hope it didn't happen. Now I try to deal with it more, I think. I know it is going to happen, so I am going to do something about it to try and make it go, to improve it.

I feel I am doing something to put this right, and I like to have something to get my teeth into. I don't like sort of thinking 'Well, it might be all right and it might not.' I have really got to try to do it.

Indeed, for some people the psychological aspects of therapy were the initial motivation for participation, and the reduction in symptoms provided an unexpected bonus:

I didn't think there was a cure much, but I was hoping to perhaps even make me deal with it, the psychological side more than anything else, because I was rather afraid that it would get me down, the fact that I would never know what was going to happen, it would play on my mind . . . In point of fact, [exercise therapy] has not only made me cope with it, it has lessened it, and therefore I am not having to cope with it as much anyway.

EMOTION AND AROUSAL, BELIEFS AND BEHAVIOUR

In addition to the disorientation and disequilibrium which are the focus of exercise-based therapy, the experience of vertigo usually includes a constellation of autonomic nervous system (ANS) symptoms, ranging from cold sweating and trembling to nausea and vomiting. These symptoms can be caused or exacerbated by stress and anxiety, particularly if the anxiety results in hyperventilation (which may actually increase the dizziness itself). They may also *provoke* anxiety, either because they are misinterpreted as a sign of serious or worsening illness, or simply because they add to the unpleasantness of the experience of vertigo (see Chapter 4). Therefore the ANS symptom–anxiety arousal component of the experience of vertigo can have far-reaching effects on beliefs and life-style, leading to higher levels of fear and restriction of behaviour than would result from the sensorimotor difficulties alone, and promoting avoidance of the very activities which might facilitate adaptation (including, in some cases, completion of an exercise programme). In order to reverse this vicious cycle, two principal kinds of rehabilitation can be employed. The first consists of techniques designed to lower levels of arousal and promote control of ANS functioning, while the second addresses the misperceptions attached to ANS symptoms. These two therapeutic goals and processes are in fact closely linked, as the following discussion will reveal.

Controlling arousal

Therapies which have been used successfully to enable the individual to control arousal, hyperventilation and ANS symptoms include various relaxation techniques, education in respiration control, biofeedback, and autogenic feedback training (AFT), which is a combination of biofeedback and learned control of ANS function by means of cognitive imagery. Some of these have been recommended as part of the rehabilitation of people with vertigo (see previous section), but are rarely used and have never been systematically evaluated. However, several of these therapies *have* been assessed for their effectiveness in reducing symptoms of motion sickness. Jones *et al.* (1985) included biofeedback training in control of skin conductance levels, AFT, deep muscle relaxation training, and diaphragmatic breathing in a programme that achieved an 85 per cent success rate in enabling airsick crew to return to flying. Kemmler (1984) also cites progressive relaxation and AFT as essential elements of his programme for prevention of airsickness, while Giles and Lochridge (1985) found that diaphragmatic breathing and cue-controlled relaxation allowed 35 out of 37 student pilots to achieve complete control of their symptoms.

Programmes of this kind tend to take the pragmatic approach of combining as many forms of potentially beneficial treatment as is possible and necessary. Hence it is not possible to dissociate the effects of graduated exposure to disorienting environments (employed in all these programmes) from the impact of the various techniques for ANS symptom control. The effects of adaptation to disorienting conditions, development of control of ANS functioning, and reduction of anxiety and monitoring or reporting of ANS symptoms are confounded, as many of the authors reporting their success frankly admit. Nevertheless, Jones and Hartman (1984) state that when AFT was added to relaxation and exposure to disorienting motion, the success rate of the programme increased from 40 per cent to over 75 per cent. These authors themselves stress that AFT may reduce susceptibility partly or entirely by restoring a sense of mastery, fostering the development of coping skills, and establishing a good relationship with the therapist, rather than by actually altering arousal levels directly. This view is confirmed by the account given by one woman with vertigo of how she was helped by training in relaxation techniques:

> You need to have something to work on. You see, you are told there is nothing wrong with you, then you get up the next day and feel exactly the same as you did . . . [With therapy] it seems to fall into place, and it does give you something to work on when you start getting yourself into a state. You think, 'No, hang on a minute' and think about it, do a bit of breathing, and it brings it all back down again. You have got something that you can actively do about the symptoms then . . . [Now] when I sit at my desk, I might have a little attack, and then it will just go out of my mind, and that was the end of it. Whereas before, I think I used to sit there and brace myself for it. When it comes now I just let it go, and try and forget about it, try and breathe a bit, and it tends to be all right.

There have been attempts to distinguish the processes by which autogenic feedback training helps reduce susceptibility to motion sickness (Cowings and Toscano 1982; Toscano and Cowings 1982). These researchers claim that AFT has no effect on the perception of motion and disequilibrium, but does enhance tolerance of the unpleasant effects of making head movements during constant velocity rotation. Tolerance was higher after AFT training than when subjects endured the same motions either with no training, or while performing a cognitive task designed to distract them from their symptoms. However, Cowings presented no evidence showing that control of ANS symptoms themselves actually occurs (see also Cowings 1990). Tolerance may therefore have been enhanced by indirect mechanisms such as those suggested by Jones and Hartman (1984), although in that case it is evident that AFT can promote a greater sense of confidence or mastery than can the cognitive distraction techniques used as a control condition.

Dobie *et al.* (1987) examined tolerance of a rotating visual surround after training in the control of forehead muscle activity and hand temperature, using biofeedback. This was compared with cognitive-behavioural therapy, which included relaxation and ten sessions of 'systematic desensitisation' by exposure to rotation of a visual surround. Subjects in the biofeedback group achieved control of EMG responses, but their tolerance of visual field motion did not improve. The tolerance of subjects given the cognitive-behavioural therapy improved to an equal extent whether or not they additionally received biofeedback training. However, once again the effects of adaptation, relaxation, systematic desensitisation and cognitive therapy were confounded in the cognitive-behavioural therapy condition.

Changing perceptions and expectancies

In addition to directly reducing tension and the physiological arousal component of anxiety, training in relaxation teaches the individual an active coping technique and demonstrates that he or she has some control over unpleasant situations or states. Encouragement to explore the nature, cause and control of symptoms in a safe, therapeutic setting may lead to significant modification of beliefs that previously caused anxiety. The exploratory aspect of forms of rehabilitation intended primarily to bring about changes in sensorimotor co-ordination and skill or control of physiological functioning may thus provide the individual with an opportunity to discover vitally important information. For example, exercise therapy may reveal that the disorientation provoked by movement is self-limiting and controllable, and does not herald the onset of a full-blown attack of vertigo, and that movement-provoked symptoms are a part of the process of compensation rather than a sign of recurring illness. Similarly, while learning to recognise and control autonomic symptoms, the individual also learns that these can simply be indicators of arousal or anxiety levels, rather than signs of serious disease. In this respect, the basis for employing AFT for vertigo resembles the rationale for 'interoceptive exposure therapy', or exposure to somatic sensations, for people subject to panic attacks (e.g. Klosko et al. 1990). It is interesting to note that the vestibular sensations induced by rotation have been used as the stimulus for therapy of this type (Barlow et al. 1989).

The impact of these informational aspects of programmes of exercise therapy and training in relaxation and respiratory control is by no means undermined by the apparently 'incidental' nature of the learning process. Indeed, actively discovering the nature and limits of the experience of vertigo by means of practical exploration may be the most powerful way that an individual can acquire the information, beliefs and confidence that are needed to encourage and support the resumption of an adaptive and fulfilling life-style (Bandura 1982). Nevertheless, rehabilitation can also directly address the evaluative and intentional components of the experience of vertigo by means of cognitive and behavioural therapy. It was noted in Chapter 2 that the 'reassurance' routinely offered by health professionals is frequently insufficient to allay fears about the significance and likely consequences of symptoms. Bandura (1982) outlines four sources of information which can promote confidence: simple verbal reassurance by the doctor; detailed physiological explanations; the example provided by other patients who are recovering or coping well; and activities which encourage individuals to explore their own capabilities, such as physically challenging treadmill exercises, which demonstrate to people who have had a heart attack that they can safely undertake strenuous activity. He asserts that verbal information is the least and behavioural demonstration the most effective means of boosting self-confidence. Positive evaluations of one's own potential or actual competence, arising from personal or vicarious experiences of successful goal-directed activity, provide the motivation and confidence to continue to pursue desired goals and overcome obstacles to success (Bandura 1977). Beneficial changes in perceptions of symptoms and the ability to cope with them may therefore be achieved by deliberately exploring the parameters of these symptoms during programmes of exercise therapy. Performing movements which may induce dizziness can be thought of as a 'behavioural experiment' which demonstrates to the individual the true extent of his or her actual and potential capabilities, and thus results in revised evaluations of self-competence. My own experience has provided some (admittedly anecdotal) evidence for this. In a study of ANS symptoms associated with vertigo, I was obliged to ask people with vertigo to perform the multiple head movements that would provoke vertigo. Before doing so they were naturally apprehensive, as most had studiously avoided these movements for months or even years. However, after making the head movements many people commented, with delighted relief, that the consequences had been much less severe than they had expected.

The informational aspect of programmes of therapy can be made more explicit by focusing on the goals, difficulties and environments that are most salient to the individual concerned. For example, after competence in a range of movements and perceptual conditions has been achieved in the clinic, it may be helpful to set explicit goals and practice targets for demonstrating competence in real-life situations, such as relaxing in a busy shopping mall, or walking down an escalator (Beyts 1987). This ensures that the skills, knowledge and confidence acquired in the safe therapeutic setting are perceived as applicable to the environments encountered in daily life. Jeans and Orrell (1991) report that the near-total disability of a woman with symptoms of 'space phobia' (dizziness and fear of falling or going out) was greatly reduced by encouragement from family and therapists to gradually but systematically attempt activities which she had abandoned. The accounts of two people with vertigo whose exercise therapy was complemented by graded goal setting also indicate that this can be a useful way of pacing exposure to disorienting situations and building confidence:

> I couldn't stand any sort of movement at all when this first happened. I could only sort of stand five minutes in the car, and I just had to get out because I felt so ill . . . I could just walk to the bottom of the road, and I gradually went a bit further and further, and then I got on the bus, and I went a couple of stops, and the next week I would go a bit further, and I gradually built it up from there.

> You have to set targets, well, the first thing I had to do was write down the things that I wanted to do. Well, there's me putting 'Walking down to the Post Office' which is only down to the end of the road and to the right. But by the time I'd left [therapy] I'd done every one of my targets, which I never, ever thought I'd be able to do . . . Just walking down to [town], you know, I'm sort of wobbling as I'm going down, but by the time I've been and I'm coming back I'm feeling good because I've done it.

Certain facets of cognitive-behavioural therapy focus explicitly on exposing and exploring unrealistic fears and misperceptions, and should therefore be relevant to achieving genuine reassurance with respect to the anxieties which accompany vertigo. Some therapists start by providing the individual with general information about his or her condition and theories relating to aetiology and recovery (Klosko *et al.* 1990; Nicholas *et al.* 1991; Pearce and Erskine 1989). This stage is similar to the education about the cause, course and treatment of vertigo currently provided by health professionals, but with sufficient time provided for wide-ranging and detailed discussion. However, in cognitive therapy the individual is then encouraged to examine his or her own particular experience in order to detect specific, idiosyncratic symptoms and processes, and relevant beliefs, behaviour, and environmental factors (Barlow *et al.* 1989). Exploration can take the form of a debate with the therapist.

Changing attitudes

In a longitudinal study, people whose questionnaire responses had indicated that they were partially handicapped by vertigo (Yardley and

Putman 1992) were sent a second questionnaire six months later, and were asked to state whether they thought that either their vertigo or their ability to *cope* with vertigo had improved or deteriorated, and why. Most people reported being better able to cope and less handicapped. Some attributed their recovery to spontaneous remission or control of symptoms by drugs. However, the most common reason given for the improvement in well-being was a change in attitude. Respondents were less anxious about the causes of vertigo, and had come to terms with its effects: 'I know what to expect and not to get afraid like I used to'; 'I take every day as it comes and live life to the full'; 'I have learned to live with it, and try to ignore it'.

To a certain extent, habituation to vertigo seems to result simply from the familiarity of prolonged experience:

After a while, when you've had it so long, you sort of get used to it.

It's something I've learned to live with, it doesn't bother me as such now – I've got used to it really.

I did worry about the future in the beginning, but now it doesn't bother me in the least. I have had [vertigo] an awful long time now, and you do get used to anything, I suppose.

Some people find that the eventual provision of a diagnosis enables them to cease worrying about their condition, and to come to terms with it:

When, gradually, you know what it was, you accept the fact that you've got that particular thing wrong with you, and it don't seem quite as bad then.

You feel if there's a handle to it [i.e. diagnosis], in many ways you can deal with it better.

I think that the only way to deal with it is to put it behind me and forget about it as much as possible, or be realistic about it. I'm very determined, I mean, I try not to let it stop me doing anything if I can, I've tried not to let it worry me. I thought 'Well, at least I haven't got two horrible things [he had suspected multiple sclerosis or a brain tumour], I'm not going to die of it, so be positive.'

Others simply resolve that the best solution is to try not to anticipate the worst and to make the most of the periods which are free from illness and incapacity, as recommended in the following accounts. (Since many of the excerpts in this book were taken from interviews with people from a maritime town, examples of successful coping often seemed to revolve around the very active, disorienting and somewhat hazardous pastime of sailing!)

> Get on with life, see what happens today. It may not happen tomorrow, it may not happen for another six weeks – you've got to use the time when it's not happening to do the things you normally do, do those things you like doing. If you like sailing, to go, but to go with someone who can handle the boat, so that if anything happens there's someone there who can take over, look after the situation.

> I've started sailing again this summer, and it's the first time I've done that for years. I've taken the attitude that [the vertigo] has stopped me doing so many things that I've decided that I want to go sailing, and if I do feel bad after it, then I'll put up with it and enjoy myself while I'm sailing.

This latter statement illustrates how the paralysing dilemmas (see Chapters 4 and 5) posed by inconsistency between long-term goals, such as maintaining a normal life-style, and behaviour directed towards achieving sub-goals, such as avoiding activities that might provoke vertigo, can be resolved by consciously establishing priorities and devising acceptable compromises (Powers 1973; Scheier and Carver 1988).

Although many of the preceding accounts seem to describe a fairly easy and practical adjustment to vertigo, expressions of resolve to cope with vertigo often have a more determined, even desperate, quality:

> I sat one morning on the bed, and I thought, 'Well, if it's going to stay, you've got to make the best of it, not let it dominate you that it's there all the time.' You can't sit and think about it, you've got to get on, and I think that's what I've done.

> You've got to get used to it, otherwise . . . It ends up, you either cope with it, or else you end up staying home. So I made my mind up that it wasn't going to affect me, so it was all right after that.

In a study of people with multiple sclerosis, Pollock (1993) has observed that the theme of achieving control over illness by an effort of will dominates the discourse of people with chronic physical illness. She notes that this somewhat moralistic rhetoric, which is strongly reinforced by the family, fellow sufferers, healthy people, and health professionals alike, represents a means of exerting pressure on the sick or disabled to minimise their deviation from normal behaviour. The danger of such a rhetoric is that failure to 'fight' the illness may then be attributed to a deficiency of motivation or weakness of character.

Although this book can itself be construed as implicitly supporting the normative notion that anxious and passive reactions to vertigo are undesirable, the potentially condemnatory aspect of this discourse has been avoided by repeatedly emphasising the understandable and justifiable nature of such reactions. Moreover, as Pollock herself observes, the idea of fighting their illness is undeniably popular with sufferers, and is associated with high self-esteem. This is partly because the ideal of 'successful coping' provides sick people with a positive goal, and the opportunity to demonstrate their competence and recover a respected social identity. Indeed, it is interesting that many people specifically linked the idea that they were able to overcome their problems with 'downward comparisons' (see Chapter 5) with other people supposedly unable to achieve such control over their more severe illness:

> You can't let it rule your life, that's what I always say, it's got to be pushed away as much as possible, you can't feel sorry for yourself really – I think I'm lucky that I'm not any worse, I mean I could be arthritic or something and then not able to do anything.

> There are times, like when I'm going out and I wonder, 'Is it going to get bad?' you know, and I think, 'Oh, I mustn't think that way, I've made it so far.' So I think positive, rather than negative . . . I mean, there are times when you feel very low, and you think – well, I think – 'There's a lot of people worse off.'

ACTIVE COPING AND THE ENVIRONMENT

Despite the most energetic use of therapies of various kinds, some people will experience intermittent recurrences of vertigo, or are left with a degree of residual disorientation or imbalance. None the less, individuals who find themselves in this situation are often able to identify various ways in which their activities or environment can be adapted so as to minimise the negative impact of the vertigo on day-to-day life:

> I actually got to the stage when I thought 'Will I have to give up my job, will I have to move house?' and think those things through. We're lucky that we live in a bungalow, so I don't have stairs to contend with, and therefore I felt I couldn't damage myself. If anything happened that I couldn't drive, we would almost certainly have to move house to somewhere within easy reach of the station, or a better bus. That's one of the things I thought about when I was going

back into a job, and I thought, 'Well, at least I could probably do [computer programming] sitting down, if the worst comes to the worst.' It wasn't the sole reason why I chose the job, but it's something I thought about – that if I was stuck, and sort of couldn't get around, then it was something I could do.

As the preceding section indicates, although medical diagnosis and treatment are commonly regarded as the primary method of mastering vertigo, sufferers are not passively and uncritically dependent upon the resources and guidance offered to them by health professionals. In their attempts to understand and cope with the vertigo, many individuals informally experiment with various types and dosages of drugs, as well as with acupuncture, homeopathic remedies, diets and faith healing. Moreover, many sources of information about vertigo other than that provided by medical professionals are utilised. Some people use medical textbooks to arrive at personal decisions concerning diagnosis and treatment. Others find that fellow sufferers can provide the most pertinent advice, as well as independent, compelling confirmation of tentative insights that they had arrived at as a result of their own experiences. Indeed, in a questionnaire study of 127 people with vertigo (Yardley 1994b), 77 per cent of the sample reported that they had looked out for books, newspaper or magazine articles, or television programmes about vertigo, and 40 per cent had consulted medical textbooks on the subject. In addition, 42 per cent of the respondents reported asking friends and relatives for practical advice, while 73 per cent had tried to talk to other people with similar problems.

A range of strategies are employed by people with vertigo in order to control their condition and maintain an active, albeit slightly adapted, life-style. Some of these involve altering the way in which routine activities are performed, so as to avoid overtaxing limited perceptual-motor capabilities and exposing the individual to danger:

[on the bike] I was all right so long as I go in a straight line and no hand signals, so I didn't do any hand signals. I used to get off, and walk my bike round corners, of course not go along any main roads.

You shouldn't walk near the edge of the pavement, or a railway station, because it could happen, you know. I mean, you've got to be aware, not think of it all the time, but be aware that it may happen, and so you've got to try and keep yourself in a reasonably safe situation.

[When I have an attack] I just have to go into an office and lie down for 10 minutes, and then gradually sort of get up on my elbows, and then I sort of sit against the wall, and then sort of gently sort of rise holding on to the wall all the time.

New and ingenious ways in which common artifacts can be un-obtrusively utilised for support when necessary have been identified by some individuals:

I bought the camper van so that if we went off anywhere at least there was somewhere to sleep, and I could throw up without all and sundry looking at me.

You just feel as though you can't keep your balance when there's nothing around you, but I've got a trolley, which is a four-wheeled sort of trolley, but it's a very, very strong one, and I take that with me when I go out. I must have something, hold something in my right hand; that's my trolley (I can't hold my trolley with my left hand because I tip over to the right).

Another tactic described by people with vertigo is to wear flat shoes with thin, non-slip soles, thereby increasing the availability of useful somatosensory information and reducing the risk of a fall. Often sufferers find that the handicap resulting from vertigo can be reduced by altering characteristics of their physical and social environment. One person replaced boldly patterned wallpaper in the bedroom with neutral colour, so that the visual environment was less disorienting when lying in bed during an acute attack. A woman who was no longer able to drive started a local bus-users' group, and found that this brought appreciable social benefits.

In a rare published personal account of adapting to the experience of vertigo, Shereen Farber (1989) describes how she was able to find numerous constructive ways of altering her behaviour and environment in order to cope with Ménière's disease. In the days immediately following her first acute attack of vertigo she learned to dress without having to bend over or balance on one leg, and immediately consulted the medical literature to find out more about her condition while waiting to see the doctor. During the next few weeks she trained her dog to walk more slowly, developed a new technique for bowling which did not involve adopting a disorienting position, and rearranged the positions of her surgical instruments at work to reduce the amount of head movement required, even building a special stand for her surgical microscope. Subsequently, she deliberately adapted her behaviour again in order to assist the process of compensation and resumption of normal patterns of activity. However, Shereen Farber was aided by an occupational grounding in rehabilitative techniques, and she herself writes that

Perhaps other people also would have been able to make the necessary adaptations to their occupational activities; it is certainly true,
however, that the problem-solving skills and the creativity I
developed during my years as an occupational therapist enabled me
to rapidly adjust to the condition. Still, even with all my skills and
resources, I experienced considerable emotional strain.

(1989: 342)

Just as social factors play an important role in the handicap associated
with vertigo (see Chapter 5), adaptation can be aided by the understanding, support and example that can best be provided by either people
who are close to the individual concerned, or those who have shared
similar experiences (Bandura 1982; Beyts 1987; Pearce and Erskine
1989). The influence of the social environment can be harnessed to
enhance the benefits of therapy by encouraging the participation of the
family in the rehabilitation programme, or by organising group therapy,
which allows group members to benefit from the support, experience
and example of each other. The latter type of support can also, of course,
be found outside official programmes of therapy, in the form of self-help
groups. In the United States, the Vestibular Disorders Association
(VEDA) provides information and support to people with vertigo, and
by disseminating the names and addresses of members allows them to
share their experiences, ideas and coping strategies. In the United
Kingdom, the Ménière's Society serves a similar function (see
Appendix for addresses of these organisations). Interestingly, while
members of the Ménière's Society interviewed in the studies reported in
this book said they found the information and support it provided very
helpful, they had all learned of the society through friends and the
media, rather than from health professionals. The existence of the
society is not widely advertised in medical environments, and some
doctors express a concern that patients' fears might be exacerbated by
meeting other people who may have worse forms or experiences of the
same disorder. There have been no specific investigations to determine
whether this is a serious risk, or whether such potential costs are out-
weighed by the benefits of a self-help group. However, there is evidence
to suggest that patients generally welcome additional information about
their illness, even when this includes potentially distressing knowledge
(Ley 1988), and that awareness of people who are worse affected by
illness actually tends to boost confidence (Taylor 1983).

SUMMARY AND CONCLUSIONS

In this chapter, a wide variety of kinds of information, exploration, support and therapy have been described which each have potential or (partially) proven utility for ameliorating different features of the experience of vertigo. Drugs, surgery, and many forms of exercise or physiotherapy can help to limit disability (disorientation and disequilibrium) and to restore and enhance sensorimotor functioning. A range of relaxation techniques, coupled with deliberate, controlled exploration of feared sensations, situations, and activities, can be used to reduce anxiety and over-arousal and exorcise the exaggerated or unrealistic fears which fuel the cycle of distress and behavioural restriction. In addition, the physical and social environment can be selected or modified so as to minimise risks (ranging from instability to embarrassment) and provide information, opportunities and support, whether in the form of settings in which the demands for sensorimotor co-ordination are minimal and the individual can safely rest or recuperate, or in the shape of people who may be able to help with empathy, tips, encouragement, or supportive actions.

The preceding analysis of the processes involved in adjusting to vertigo suggests that, just as the negative elements of the experience of vertigo have multifaceted and interactive characteristics, the benefits of therapy and active coping measures may well also be multidimensional. Hence, part of the therapeutic effect of exercise programmes may emanate from the concrete demonstration that movement will not provoke unbearable and unmanageable dizziness. Similarly, the value of education in relaxation techniques may actually be that confidence is enhanced by the acquisition of an active coping skill. Conversely, encouragement to experience feared sensations or resume feared activities (using methods of 'graded exposure' or 'systematic desensitisation') may have physical benefits, by providing the learning opportunities needed for central compensation and the development of sensorimotor co-ordination and skill.

Although this chapter provides an analysis of the potential usefulness of various forms of information, therapy and support, further research is needed in order systematically to evaluate the *actual* relative value of each therapy. For example, to date there have been no properly conducted, randomised comparisons of the various drug therapies with different exercise programmes, nor of physiotherapy with cognitive-behavioural therapy and autogenic feedback training. Moreover, quite apart from the methodological failings of the clinical trials detailed in the preceding sections of this chapter, important questions concerning how the mutual effects of various *combinations* of therapies might enhance (or hinder) rehabilitative processes have scarcely been investigated in the context of vertigo. Hence, it is unknown whether relaxation training or cognitive therapy might increase compliance with exercise programmes by providing the individual with a method of coping with the frightening sensations provoked by exercises, or whether behavioural therapy might be usefully combined with exercises in order to ensure that improvement in physical capabilities and confidence generalises to behaviour outside the therapeutic environment. It is to be hoped that future developments in rehabilitation will seek to understand, address and exploit the complex reciprocal processes which contribute both to the maintenance and escalation of handicap, and to adjustment and habituation to vertigo.

Chapter 7

Concluding comments
Towards a new approach to disorientation

Looking back over the analyses of various aspects of the experience of vertigo presented in this book, the gradual emergence of three interrelated themes can be discerned, introducing a fresh perspective on the subject of disorientation. The fact that these new ways of conceptualising the problem of vertigo and dizziness were to a large extent arrived at empirically, and are firmly grounded in the details of the accounts and analyses which gave rise to them, is a key feature of their claim to value and validity. None the less, the principles derived from an intensive study of vertigo have the potential to extend our understanding not only of disorientation, but also of a host of complex chronic disorders which share many essential characteristics with the experience of vertigo.

The first theme relates to the fundamentally multidimensional nature of vertigo, which is portrayed as the dynamic product of reciprocal interactions between somatic symptoms and psychological predispositions, activities and their environmental context, beliefs and their behavioural and physiological consequences. The term 'multidimensional' is thus intended not only to convey the many-faceted nature of vertigo, but also to advance a dimensional rather than a categorical view of the factors contributing to disorientation, and an accent on processes rather than static traits or properties. These implicit features of the multidimensional approach themselves give rise to the second theme: namely, replacement of the traditional conception of the 'patient–sufferer' as the passive victim of disease by one of the individual who actively contributes to the experience of vertigo, not only constructing meaning from the confusion and uncertainty that is intrinsic to disorientation and adapting his or her life-style to the illness, but thereby actually influencing the nature and course of symptoms and disability. The third theme concerns the impact of context on the experience of vertigo, both in terms of the immediate physical and social environment, and the broader socio-cultural context which provides the framework within which vertigo is understood. These new perspectives on disorientation should foster an appreciation of the contribution of non-pathological factors to the experience, suggest promising topics for research, and pave the way for innovative approaches to therapy.

THE MULTIDIMENSIONAL NATURE OF VERTIGO

The multiplicity of the elements which contribute to vertigo is repeatedly emphasised and quite comprehensively covered by this book; indeed, each section of every chapter details the relevance of a distinct component of the experience of vertigo, from the uncertainties surrounding diagnosis to the potential benefits of self-help groups. The novelty in this approach does not derive from the nature or diversity of the topics covered; the way in which illness affects and is affected by family relationships, medical discourse, attributions, or psychophysiological processes are not new topics for discussion, although no overview of these aspects of vertigo and dizziness in particular has previously been undertaken. However, despite the increasing popularity of a systemic 'biopsychosocial' approach to illness (Engel 1977; Schwartz 1982), few authors until now have attempted a truly integrated analysis of the physiological, cognitive, behavioural, environmental and socio-cultural aspects of a particular condition. Indeed, the distinction between the biomedical and psychosocial features of an ailment is often maintained as enthusiastically by social scientists affirming the primacy of the psychosocial construction of 'the illness experience' as by medical scientists asserting the primacy of organic disease. In contrast, this book depicts the experience of vertigo as indivisible, in that *interactions* between the organic, psychological and environmental features of the condition fashion the immediate and long-term effects on physiological, functional and psychosocial processes.

Adoption of a truly multidimensional approach to disorientation has several implications for the investigation and treatment of vertigo. First, it demands a rejection of the traditional medical view of the organic disease as central, and the various functional and psychosocial aspects as merely epiphenomena. Within the medical model, behavioural, cognitive and emotional aspects of vertigo have traditionally been treated as isolable from the fundamental condition; for sound diagnostic reasons every effort is made to distinguish between physical as opposed to mental disturbance, difficult though this often proves to be. Concomitant psychological disorders have therefore been proposed as an explanation for the well-documented 'desynchrony' between objective estimates of physical pathology and subjective patient complaints (Hallam *et al.* 1988). Factors such as hypothetical predisposing personality traits, stress, or the 'psychogenic' contribution to complaints of vertigo, are treated as independent from and potentially obscuring or distracting from the underlying disease, and are relegated to the realm of psychiatry (or clinical psychology).

This book has sought to demonstrate that while the sharp distinction between physical and psychical, 'normal' and pathological, may be important to the diagnosis and management of organic disease, it is a somewhat arbitrary distinction in terms of human experience. Moreover, once the role of reciprocal interactions between different features of the experience of dizziness is recognised, it is clear that restriction of the scope of enquiry and treatment to physical pathology is bound to limit their effectiveness, whether assessed in narrow biomedical terms or according to broader criteria such as biopsychosocial well-being or quality of life. A multidimensional approach reveals that the context – psychological, environmental and social – crucially determines the nature and consequences of the physical component of a balance system disorder. Hence an appreciation of these aspects of disorientation is requisite not only for an understanding of the links between vertigo, anxiety and handicap, but also in order to interpret the results of tests for balance system impairment, predict the circumstances that will trigger an episode of vertigo, or design a treatment programme that can successfully promote neurophysiological compensation. But while levels of analysis other than the pathophysiological must be recognised as of central importance to the understanding and management of disorientation, it is equally vital to avoid the mistake of 'psychologising' the illness (Goudsmit and Gadd 1991). Physical symptoms and physiological changes constitute the foundation for the psychosocial experience of illness, both directly and indirectly influencing attitudes, emotions, behaviour and social relationships (Kirmayer 1992).

THE ROLE OF ACTIVITY

An implicit characteristic of a systemic biopsychosocial approach is that the conception of the experience of illness as created by reciprocal interactions between diverse elements militates against unidirectional models of causation. The multidimensional approach to disorientation thus bypasses the debate about cause and effect in the relationship between vertigo and psychological characteristics, and seeks instead to explain the complex interactions between disease, disability, beliefs and behaviour in terms of meaningful human activity. From this perspective, it is inappropriate to consider individuals as the passive victims either of internal physical or psychological pathology, or of external stresses or insults. The impact of internal and external disturbances can only be understood in the context of the previous experiences, current activities and subsequent goals and intentions of the individual, set in the broader context of his or her environment. The individual, whether healthy or not, is consequently viewed as a purposeful, adaptive human being acting within a particular environmental context. This description of the person with vertigo opens up a number of formerly neglected topics for exploration; for example, examination of the physiological, perceptual and social consequences of changes in goals, activities and ways of interacting with the environment. The individual's active role in the creation and maintenance of the experience of vertigo thus itself becomes an important new subject for investigation. Examples in this book include the analysis of how self-generated rules for coping with vertigo may lead to anticipatory disability, and of how skills and strategies may contribute to perceptual-motor adaptation.

Awareness of the importance of activity introduces an emphasis on processes rather than traits, and this may also influence the way in which people with vertigo are construed. When medical prognoses and cures are unavailable, diagnostic classification can be reduced to the ascription of somewhat static and unproductive labels. Patients are described in terms of abnormal properties or categories; they have 'vertigo', 'Ménière's disease', 'neurotic personality traits' or 'panic disorder', or may even *be* 'a case of vestibular neuronitis' or 'an agoraphobic'. In contrast, a process-oriented approach avoids premature evaluation of the condition of someone experiencing disorientation as necessarily either immutable or even abnormal; anxiety may be a rational response to a poorly understood threat, while symptoms of vertigo may be amenable to reinterpretation and adaptive management. Hence, a focus on process provides an escape from the unproductive and possibly damaging discourses which centre on reductionist and dualistic distinctions between mind and body, the normal and the pathological.

An appreciation of how people with vertigo actively adapt to their situation in an effort to maintain a meaningful and viable life-style contrasts with the tendency of traditional medicine to treat the patient as a passive battleground upon which the doctor conducts surgical and chemical warfare against the disease. Recognition of the active participation of the sick individual consequently has significant implications for rehabilitation. Since the individual plays a central role in constructing his or her personal experience of vertigo, he or she should also be capable of dispelling or avoiding many of the negative aspects of this experience. Accordingly, the task of the health professional should not be to 'administer' treatment, 'manage' the patient, or 'control' the vertigo, but rather to facilitate the individual's attempts to adapt by providing the necessary information, training, skills and support – whether social, psychological, practical, or medical.

A number of benefits may be gained by encouraging increased participation of the patient in the process of coping with vertigo. First, it is evident from many of the comments and findings included in this book that patients desire, and often informally seek, a more active and informed role in self-care than that routinely offered to them. Encouraging active participation in management of the vertigo is likely to enhance the confidence and self-reliance of patients with respect to coping with illness. In addition, while an exclusively therapist-controlled approach to treatment can certainly achieve beneficial results, it places an enormous burden of responsibility on the therapist, who must identify precisely which forms of treatment are needed by a particular patient at each stage of his or her rehabilitation, with minimal formal assistance from the individual concerned. If the necessary elements of rehabilitation are not correctly identified then interventions will be incompletely successful. For example, medication may prove able to limit the recurrence of acute attacks of vertigo but fail to clear up residual dizziness, while a programme of exercises may restore normal balance function without addressing the problem of lasting fear and avoidance of certain real-life activities or environments. Moreover, without the understanding and active participation of the individual with vertigo, the treatment programme may not be properly followed. To take just two instances I have encountered in the course of my clinical work, medication designed for symptomatic control (e.g. vestibular sedatives) may be mistaken for a prophylactic and come to be relied upon for prevention of attacks, thus preventing complete central compensation, while drugs prescribed because of putative long-term preventative or curative effects may be taken, ineffectively, to treat acute symptoms. On a day-to-day basis, it is the individual with vertigo, and not the clinician, who must instigate, monitor, and ultimately achieve adjustment to the illness and control of its unpleasant consequences. Hence, by encouraging the patient to adopt an active, informed, problem-solving role, it may be possible to attain those unique, fine-tuned adaptations to the experience of vertigo that only the individual concerned can identify, initiate, and implement.

A final consideration motivating promotion of a more active patient role is the fact that the expertise and resources of health professionals are both costly and finite. Consequently, there is a need to attempt to enhance the scope and effectiveness of health care by enlisting the active participation of the individual concerned in the process of diagnosis and rehabilitation. If people with vertigo themselves can become expert in the skills of monitoring, discriminating and evaluating symptoms and provoking factors, and developing and testing appropriate behavioural adaptations and modifications to the environment, then they may be better able to cope in the long term without professional help. Hence, despite the obstacles posed by patients' expectations of a rapid and effortless cure, and health professionals' reluctance to allocate the necessary time to provision of information and training, the lasting benefits that might be achieved by promoting informed self-care may merit the time and effort this demands.

THE CONTEXT OF DISORIENTATION

This book has repeatedly illustrated how the physical, social and biographical context of an individual can profoundly influence his or her experience of vertigo: a family history of central nervous system disease may enhance fears of serious illness and the desire for medical investigation and reassurance; a physically hazardous job and unsympathetic employer can result in greatly increased levels of handicap; encounters with disorienting man-made environments may trigger disconcerting episodes of unexpected dizziness. From the preoccupation with the social impact of dizziness evident in the accounts given in this book, the social context of disorientation appears especially salient. The attitudes of confidants and strangers, friends and colleagues strongly affect the outlook, behaviour and well-being of people with vertigo, sometimes supporting the process of adjustment, but sometimes adding to the cycle of isolation, inactivity and impotence that can accompany vertigo.

Consideration of the role of context provides a further rationale for ensuring that the person with vertigo is an active participant in the medical consultation. Herzlich (1973) has observed how, from the time that we first play 'doctors and patients' as children, the doctor–patient relationship teaches the individual the attitudes and behaviour expected by society from and towards someone who is ill. The context of a real consultation thus to some extent acts as a microcosm of the social world, on the basis of which patients may infer the normative social attitudes pertaining to their condition and learn to rehearse the normative behaviour and discourse. Hence, if the priority given to biomedical diagnosis and treatment leads health professionals to minimise, ignore or dismiss the beliefs and concerns of people with vertigo, sufferers are likely to conclude that their condition is inherently stigmatising and even less likely to receive understanding and sympathetic treatment from people with no knowledge of vertigo. Similarly, if patients are excluded from the relevant information, decisions and responsibility, they will also conclude that they are ignorant and powerless to deal with the problem, and may well adopt a correspondingly helpless 'sick role'. In contrast, if the observations, hypotheses, and anxieties of these individuals regarding the aetiology, course and treatment of their illness are taken seriously, they are more likely to perceive the illness as no obstacle to maintaining a competent, self-respecting social role and image.

In this book, examination of the role of context has been restricted to a consideration of the immediate, personal context of the individual. However, the way in which the broader socio-economic, -linguistic, -cultural and -historical context shapes the immediate context of disorientation constitutes a fascinating and potentially valuable topic for future analysis. For example, while the intellectual origins of the physical–psychological distinction which has obstructed the development of a biopsychosocial approach to dizziness can be traced to the mind–body dualism inherent in the western Cartesian philosophical tradition, the physical manifestation of this tradition is embodied in the separate disciplines and professions of psychiatry and neurology, psychology and physiology. Since members of each profession tend to operate independently from each other, and often seem to offer competing rather than co-operative explanations and remedies for disorientation, this living intellectual tradition can have an enormous influence on the experience of people with vertigo. Referral of people with disorientation to a psychiatrist or psychologist will result in detailed exploration of their feelings and fears, and perhaps even an enquiry into the symbolic meanings associated with their disorientation, but the perceptual-motor factors which may be contributing to their problems and the possibility of physical rehabilitation will probably be overlooked. Similarly, those referred to neuro-otologists or audio-vestibular clinicians will receive rigorous physical examination, investigation and treatment of balance system dysfunction, but will be offered only limited help with the psychosocial problems which so often accompany vertigo.

Finally, examination of the discourses which are employed to articulate the experience and perception of vertigo, and the way these are shaped by context, may prove illuminating. Radley (1993) has illustrated how people who are ill may use transfiguring metaphors to escape the useless and painful oscillation between literal hope and despair. This imaginative construction of a new reality which can incorporate and transcend the illness parallels the therapeutic 'experiencing' which Vasilyuk (1991) suggests must mediate adjustment to a painful situation which is not amenable to practical resolution. Radley is at pains to emphasise that the use of metaphor to adjust to illness is not a private affair, since the power and legitimacy of a metaphor lies partly in its reference to acceptable ideologies and social relationships. The prevalent attitudes towards disorientation within society are therefore bound to affect the process of personal adaptation. For example, Herzlich (1973) has suggested that people with chronic illness progress from a 'destructive' perspective, from which illness is seen as alien and deviant, to an acceptance of the struggle against illness as a form of socially valid activity, and notes that an informed and active collaboration with the doctor is a necessary condition for adoption of the latter, positive social role. Yet this role may be effectively denied to individuals who feel that their position is undermined by tacit suspicions, or at least connotations, of emotional weakness and hypochondria. It seems likely that the common ambivalent attitudes relating to the validity of dizziness as a physical ailment will therefore delay acceptance and adjustment; the sufferer cannot proceed to the socially normative and rewarding task of successfully coping with illness until its authenticity has been confirmed by doctors and acknowledged by family, friends, employers and colleagues.

The scope of this book has been much broader than any other on the topic, incorporating aspects of the problem of vertigo which have seldom or never hitherto been considered. However, it has been devoted almost exclusively to analysis of interactions between the individual and his or her immediate context. The cultural practices and social constraints which, for instance, inhibit adults from relearning balancing skills or strongly encourage attempts to cope with illness have been mentioned in passing, but it was beyond the remit of this book to embark on a more thorough discussion of the origins of a rhetoric of rationality or control with regard to emotions and illness, or to examine how moralistic psychosomatic theories may also serve as 'legends which hint at the transcendental side of all our suffering' (Guggenbühl-Craig and Micklem 1988: 146). In order to extend and deepen our understanding of disorientation, future investigations should therefore look beyond this somewhat localised and rationalist focus, to explore the hidden assumptions, myths and purposes behind the discourses which establish the meaning of disorientation in society.

Appendix

VESTIBULAR DISORDERS ASSOCIATION
PO Box 4467,
Portland,
Oregon 97208–4467
USA

MÉNIÈRE'S SOCIETY
98 Maybury Road,
Woking,
Surrey GU21 5HX
UK

References

Abramson, L. Y., Seligman, M. E. P. and Teasdale, J. D. (1978). Learned helplessness in humans: critique and reformulation. *Journal of Abnormal Psychology, 87*, 49–74.

Allum, J. H. J. and Pfaltz, C. R. (1985). Visual and vestibular contributions to pitch sway stabilization in the ankle muscles of normals and patients with bilateral vestibular deficits. *Experimental Brain Research, 58*, 82–94.

Allum, J. H. J., Keshner, E. A., Honegger, F. and Pfaltz, C. R. (1988). Indicators of the influence a peripheral vestibular deficit has on vestibulo-spinal reflex responses controlling postural stability. *Acta Otolaryngologica, 106*, 252–263.

Allum, J. H. J., Ura, M., Honegger, F. and Pfaltz, C. R. (1991). Classification of peripheral and central (pontine infarction) vestibular deficits: selection of a neuro-otological test battery using discriminant analysis. *Acta Otolaryngologica, 111*, 16–26.

Anderson, R. and Bury, M. (1988). *Living with Chronic Illness.* London: Unwin Hyman.

Arenberg, I. K. and Stahle, J. (1980). Staging Ménière's disease (or any inner ear dysfunction) and the use of the vertigogram. *Otolaryngologic Clinics of North America, 13*, 643–656.

Argyle, M. (1992). Benefits produced by supportive social relationships. In H. O. F. Veiel and V. Baumann (eds) *The Meaning and Measurement of Social Support.* New York: Hemisphere Publishing.

Austin, J. (1992). *Ménière's disease: the psychological aspects of the condition, with particular reference to coping and locus of control.* Unpublished M.Sc. thesis: University of Exeter.

Baddeley, A. D. (1986). *Working Memory.* Oxford: Oxford University Press.

Baddeley, A. D. and Lieberman, K. (1980). Spatial working memory. In R. S. Nickerson (ed.) *Attention and Performance, Vol. VIII.* Hillsdale, N.J.: Lawrence Erlbaum.

Bägger-Sjöbäck, D. (1988). Surgical treatment of vertigo. *Acta Otolaryngologica, 455 (Suppl.)*, 86–89.

Ballantyne, J. C. and Ajodhia, J. M. (1984). Iatrogenic dizziness. In M. R. Dix and J. D. Hood (eds) *Vertigo.* Chichester: Wiley.

Baloh, R. W. (1992). Dizziness in older people. *Journal of the American Geriatric Society, 40*, 713-721.

Baloh, R. W. and Honrubia, V. (1990). *Clinical Neurophysiology of the Vestibular System* (2nd edn). Philadelphia, PA: F. A. Davis.

Baloh, R. W., Honrubia, V. and Jacobson, K. (1987). Benign positional vertigo: clinical and oculographic features in 240 cases. *Neurology, 37*, 371–378.

Bandura, A. (1977). Self-efficacy: toward a unifying theory of behavioural change. *Psychological Review, 84*, 191–215.

Bandura, A. (1982). Self-efficacy mechanism in human agency. *American Psychologist, 37*, 122–147.

Barber, H. O. (1983). Ménière's disease: symptomatology. In W. J. Oosterveld (ed.) *Ménière's Disease: a Comprehensive Appraisal*. Chichester: Wiley.

Barlow, D. H., Craske, M. G., Cerny, J. A. and Klosko, J. S. (1989). Behavioral treatment of panic disorder. *Behavior Therapy, 20*, 261–282.

Bass, C. (1990). *Somatization*. Oxford: Blackwell Scientific Publications.

Baumann, L. J., Cameron, L. D., Zimmerman, R. S. and Leventhal, H. (1989). Illness representations and matching labels with symptoms. *Health Psychology, 8*, 449–469.

Beck, A. T. and Clark, D. A. (1991). Anxiety and depression: an information processing perspective. In R. Schwarzer and R. A. Wicklund (eds) *Anxiety and Self-focused Attention*. London: Harwood Academic Publishers.

Benson, A. J. (1984). Motion sickness. In M. R. Dix and J. D. Hood (eds) *Vertigo*. Chichester: Wilcy.

Beyts, J. P. (1987). Vestibular rehabilitation. In D. Stephens (ed.) *Adult Audiology, Scott-Brown's Otolaryngology (5th edn)*. London: Butterworths.

Black, F. O. and Nashner, L. M. (1984a). Postural disturbance in patients with benign paroxysmal positional vertigo. *Annals of Otology, Rhinology and Laryngology, 93*, 595–599.

Black, F. O. and Nashner, L. M. (1984b). Vestibulo-spinal control differs in patients with reduced versus distorted vestibular function. *Acta Otolaryngologica, 406 (Suppl.)*, 110–114.

Black, F. O., Shupert, C. L., Peterka, R. J. and Nashner, L. M. (1989). Effects of unilateral loss of vestibular function on the vestibulo-ocular reflex and postural control. *Annals of Otology, Rhinology and Laryngology, 98*, 884–889.

Bles, W., Kapteyn, T. S., Brandt, T. and Arnold, F. (1980). The mechanism of physiological height vertigo II. Posturography. *Acta Otolaryngologica, 89*, 534–540.

Bles, W. and van Raay, J. L. (1988). Pre- and post-flight postural control in tilting environments. *Advances in Oto-Rhino-Laryngology, 42*, 13–17.

Blythe, P. and McGlown, D. (1982). Agoraphobia. *World Medicine*, July, 57–59.

Brackmann, D. E. (1983). Ménière's disease: surgical treatment. In W. J. Oosterveld (ed.) *Ménière's Disease: a Comprehensive Appraisal*. Chichester: Wiley.

Brandt, T. (1984). Visual vertigo and acrophobia. In M. R. Dix and J. D. Hood (eds) *Vertigo*. Chichester: Wiley.

Brandt, T. (1991). *Vertigo: its Multisensory Syndromes*. London: Springer-Verlag.

Brandt, T., Arnold, F., Bles, W. and Kapteyn, T. S. (1980). The mechanism of physiological height vertigo I. Theoretical approach and psychophysics. *Acta Otolaryngologica, 89*, 513–523.

Brandt, T. and Daroff, R. B. (1979). The multisensory physiological and pathological vertigo syndromes. *Annals of Neurology, 7*, 195–203.

Brightwell, D. R. and Abramson, M. (1975). Personality characteristics in patients with vertigo. *Archives of Otolaryngologica, 101*, 364–366.

Brookes, G. B., Gresty, M. A., Nakamura, T. and Metcalfe, T. (1993). Sensing and controlling rotational orientation in normal subjects and patients with loss of labyrinthine function. *American Journal of Otology, 14*, 349–351.

Browning, G. G. (1986). *Clinical Otology and Audiology.* London: Butterworths.

Browning, G. G. (1991). Medical treatment for vertigo. In J. D. Hood and L. M. Goeting (eds) *Current Approaches to Vertigo*. Dorchester: Duphar.

Challis, G. B. and Stam, H. J. (1992). A longitudinal study of the development of anticipatory nausea and vomiting in cancer chemotherapy patients: the role of absorption and autonomic perception. *Health Psychology, 11*, 181–189.

Cioffi, D. (1991). Beyond attentional strategies: a cognitive-perceptual model of somatic interpretation. *Psychological Bulletin, 109*, 25–41.

Clark, D. M. (1986). A cognitive approach to panic. *Behaviour, Research and Therapy, 24*, 461–470.

Cohen, S. (1992). Stress, social support and disorder. In H. O. F. Veiel and V. Baumann (eds) *The Meaning and Measurement of Social Support*. New York: Hemisphere Publishing.

Cohn, T. E. and Lasley, D. J. (1990). Wallpaper illusion: cause of disorientation and falls on escalators. *Perception, 19*, 573–580.

Coker, N. J., Coker, R. R., Jenkins, H. A. and Vincent, K. R. (1989). Psychological profile of patients with Ménière's disease. *Archives of Otolaryngology – Head and Neck Surgery, 115*, 1355–1357.

Cooper, C. W. (1993). Vestibular neuronitis: a review of a common cause of vertigo in general practice. *British Journal of General Practice, 43*, 164–167.

Corballis, M. C. and McLaren, R. (1982). Interaction between perceived and imagined rotation. *Journal of Experimental Psychology: Human Perception and Performance, 8*, 215–224.

Corbin, J. and Strauss, A. (1985). Managing chronic illness at home: three lines of work. *Qualitative Sociology, 8*, 224–227.

Cowings, P. S. (1990). Autogenic feedback training: a treatment for motion and space sickness. In G. H. Crampton (ed.) *Motion and Space Sickness*. Boca Raton, Fla: CRC Press.

Cowings, P. S. and Toscano, W. B. (1982). The relationship of motion sickness susceptibility to learned autonomic control for symptom suppression. *Aviation, Space and Environmental Medicine, 53*, 570–575.

Coyne, J. C. and Fiske, V. (1992). Couples coping with chronic and catastrophic illness. In T. J. Akamatsu, M. A. P. Stephens, S. E. Hobfoll and J. H. Crowther (eds) *Family Health Psychology*. Washington, DC: Hemisphere Publishing Corporation.

Crampton, G. H. (ed.) (1990). *Motion and Space Sickness*. Boca Raton, Fla: CRC Press.

Crary, W. G. and Wexler, M. (1977). Ménière's disease: a psychosomatic disorder? *Psychological Reports, 41*, 603–645.

Crémieux, J. and Mesure, S. (1990). The effects of judo training on postural control assessed by accelerometry. In T. Brandt, W. Paulus, W. Bles, M.

Dieterich, S. Krafczyk and A. Straube (eds) *Disorders of Posture and Gait.* New York: Georg Thieme Verlag Stuttgart.

Crits-Christoph, P. and Mintz, J. (1991). Implications of therapist effects for the design and analysis of comparative studies of psychotherapies. *Journal of Consulting and Clinical Psychology, 59,* 20–26.

Crowley, J. S. (1987). Simulator sickness: a problem for army aviation. *Aviation, Space and Environmental Medicine, 58,* 355–357.

Crown, S. and Crisp, A. H. (1979). *Manual of the Crown–Crisp Experiential Index.* London: Hodder & Stoughton.

Cyr, D. G., Möller, C. G. and Moore, G. F. (1989). Clinical experience with the low-frequency rotary chair test. *Seminars in Hearing, 10,* 172–189.

de Jong, J. M. B. V. and Bles, W. (1986). Cervical dizziness and ataxia. In W. Bles and T. Brandt (eds) *Disorders of Posture and Gait.* Amsterdam: Elsevier.

Derogatis, L. R., Lipman, R. S., Rickels, K., Uhlenhuth, E. H. and Covi, L. (1974). The Hopkins Symptom Checklist (HSCL): a self-report symptom inventory. *Behavioral Science, 19,* 1–15.

Dichgans, J. and Diener, H.-C. (1989). The contribution of vestibulo-spinal mechanisms to the maintenance of human upright posture. *Acta Otolaryngologica, 107,* 338–345.

Dix, M. R. (1984a). The clinical examination and pharmacological treatment of vertigo. In M. R. Dix and J. D. Hood (eds) *Vertigo.* Chichester: Wiley.

Dix, M. R. (1984b). Rehabilitation of vertigo. In M. R. Dix and J. D. Hood (eds) *Vertigo.* Chichester: Wiley.

Dix, M. R. and Harrison, M. S. (1984). Positional vertigo. In M. R. Dix and J. D. Hood (eds) *Vertigo.* Chichester: Wiley.

Dix, M. R. and Hood, J. D. (eds) (1984). *Vertigo.* Chichester: Wiley.

Dobie, T. G., May, J. G., Fischer, W. D., Elder, S. T. and Kubitz, K. A. (1987). A comparison of two methods of training resistance to visually-induced motion sickness. *Aviation, Space and Environmental Medicine, 58 (Suppl.),* A34–A41.

Dowd, P. J. and Cramer, R. L. (1971). Relationship of pentathlon sports skills to vestibulo-ocular responses to coriolis stimulation. *Aerospace Medicine, 42,* 956–958.

Drachman, D. A. and Hart, C. W. (1972). An approach to the dizzy patient. *Neurology, 22,* 323–334.

DSM-III: Diagnostic and Statistical Manual of Mental Disorders (3rd edn) (1987). Washington, DC: American Psychiatric Association.

Eagger, S., Luxon, L. M., Davies, R. A., Coelho, A. and Ron, M. A. (1992). Psychiatric morbidity in patients with peripheral vestibular disorder: a clinical and neuro-otological study. *Journal of Neurology, Neurosurgery and Psychiatry, 55,* 383–387.

Engel, G. L. (1977). The need for a new medical model: a challenge for biomedicine. *Science, 196,* 129–136.

Eysenck, M. W. (1987). Trait theories of anxiety. In J. Strelau and H. J. Eysenck (eds) *Personality Dimensions and Arousal.* New York: Plenum Press.

Eysenck, M. W. (1991). Anxiety and attention. In R. Schwarzer and R. A. Wicklund (eds) *Anxiety and Self-focused Attention.* London: Harwood Academic Publishers.

Farber, S. D. (1989). Living with Ménière's disease – an occupational therapist's perspective. *American Journal of Occupational Therapy, 43,* 341–343.

Fitzpatrick, R. (1984a). Satisfaction with health care. In R. Fitzpatrick, J. Hinton, S. Newman, G. Scambler and J. Thompson (eds) *The Experience of Illness.* London: Tavistock.

Fitzpatrick, R. (1984b). Lay concepts of illness. In R. Fitzpatrick, J. Hinton, S. Newman, G. Scambler and J. Thompson (eds) *The Experience of Illness.* London: Tavistock.

Fukuda, T. (1975). Postural behaviour and motion sickness. *Acta Otolaryngologica, 330 (Suppl.),* 9–14.

Giles, D. A. and Lochridge, G. K. (1985). Behavioural airsickness management program for student pilots. *Aviation, Space and Environmental Medicine, 56,* 991–994.

Giorgi, A. (1977). The implications of Merleau-Ponty's thesis of 'The primacy of perception' for perceptual research in psychology. *Journal of Phenomenological Psychology, 8,* 81–102.

Goffman, E. (1963). *Stigma: Notes on the Management of a Spoiled Identity.* Englewood Cliffs, NJ: Prentice-Hall.

Goudsmit, E. M. and Gadd, R. (1991). All in the mind? The psychologisation of illness. *The Psychologist, 4,* 449–453.

Gray, M. (1983). Communicating with elderly people. In D. Pendleton and J. Hasler (eds) *Doctor–Patient Communication.* London: Academic Press.

Graybiel, A. (1969). Structural elements in the concept of motion sickness. *Aerospace Medicine, 40,* 351–367.

Graybiel, A., Kennedy, R. S., Knoblock, E. C., Guedry, F. E., Mertz, W., McLeod, M. E., Colehour, M. S., Miller, E. F. and Fregly, A. R. (1965). Effects of exposure to a rotating environment (10rpm) on four aviators for a period of twelve days. *Aerospace Medicine, 36,* 733–754.

Graybiel, A. and Lackner, J. R. (1980). A sudden-stop vestibulovisual test for rapid assessment of motion sickness manifestations. *Aviation, Space and Environmental Medicine, 51,* 21–23.

Green, J. D., Shelton, C. and Brackmann, D. E. (1992). Middle Fossa vestibular neurectomy in retrolabyrinthine neurectomy failures. *Archives of Otolaryngology – Head and Neck Surgery, 118,* 1058–1060.

Grimm, R. J., Hemenway, W. G., Lebray, P. R. and Black, F. O. (1989). The perilymph fistula syndrome defined in mild head trauma. *Acta Otolaryngologica, 464 (Suppl.),* 1–40.

Grisby, J. P. and Johnston, C. L. (1989). Depersonalization, vertigo and Ménière's disease. *Psychological Reports, 64,* 527–534.

Gruman, J. C. and Sloan, R. P. (1983). Disease as justice: perceptions of the victims of physical illness. *Basic and Applied Social Psychology, 4,* 39–46.

Guggenbühl-Craig, A. and Micklem, N. (1988). No answer to Job: reflections on the limitations of meaning in illness. In M. Kidel and S. Rowe-Leete (eds) *The Meaning of Illness.* London: Routledge.

Hallam, R. S. (1976). The Eysenck personality scales: stability and change after therapy. *Behaviour, Research and Therapy, 14,* 369–372.

Hallam, R. S., Beyts, J. and Jakes, S. C. (1988). Symptom reporting and objective test results: explorations of desynchrony. In S. D. G. Stephens and

S. Prasansuk (eds) *Advances in Audiology, Vol. 5: Measurement in Hearing and Balance*. Basel: Karger.

Hallam, R. S. and Hinchcliffe, R. (1991). Emotional stability: its relationship to confidence in maintaining balance. *Journal of Psychosomatic Research, 35*, 421–430.

Hallam, R. S. and Stephens, S. D. G. (1985). Vestibular disorder and emotional distress. *Journal of Psychosomatic Research, 29*, 407–413.

Hanson, M. R. (1989). The dizzy patient: a practical approach to management. *Postgraduate Medicine, 85*, 99–108.

Harris, T. O. (1992). Some reflections on the process of social support and nature of unsupportive behaviors. In H. O. F. Veiel and V. Baumann (eds) *The Meaning and Measurement of Social Support*. New York: Hemisphere Publishing.

Hauser, S. T. (1981). Physician–patient relationships. In E. G. Mishler, L. R. Amarasingham, S. D. Osherson, N. E. Waxter and R. Liem (eds) *Social Contexts of Health, Illness and Patient Care*. Cambridge: Cambridge University Press.

Häusler, R. and Pampurik, J. (1989). Surgical and physiotherapeutic treatment of the benign paroxysmal positional vertigo. *Laryngorhinootologie, 68*, 349–354.

Haye, R. and Quist-Hanssen, Sv. (1976). The natural course of Ménière's disease. *Acta Otolaryngologica, 82*, 289–293.

Hecker, H. C., Haug, C. O. and Herndon, J. W. (1974). Treatment of the vertiginous patient using Cawthorne's vestibular exercises. *The Laryngoscope, 84*, 2065–2072.

Herbst, G. and Humphrey, C. (1981). Prevalence of hearing impairment in the elderly living at home. *Journal of the Royal College of General Practitioners*, March, 155–160.

Herdman, S. J. (1990). Treatment of benign paroxysmal positional vertigo. *Physical Therapy, 70*, 381–388.

Herzlich, C. (1973). *Health and Illness*. London: Academic Press.

Hettinger, L. J., Kennedy, R. S. and McCauley, M. E. (1990). Motion and human performance. In G. H. Crampton (ed.) *Motion and Space Sickness*. Boca Raton, Fla: CRC Press.

Hinchcliffe, R. (1967). Personality profile in Ménière's disease. *Journal of Laryngology and Otology, 81*, 477–481.

Hinchcliffe, R. (1983). Psychological and sociological facets of balance disorders. In R. Hinchcliffe (ed.) *Hearing and Balance in the Elderly*. Edinburgh: Churchill Livingstone.

Hood, J. D. (1970). The clinical significance of vestibular habituation. *Advances of Oto-Rhino-Laryngology, 17*, 149–157.

Hood, J. D. (1984). Tests of vestibular function. In M. R. Dix and J. D. Hood (eds) *Vertigo*. Chichester: Wiley.

Horak, F. B., Jones-Rycewicz, C., Black, F. O. and Shumway-Cook, A. (1992). Effects of vestibular rehabilitation on dizziness and imbalance. *Otolaryngology – Head and Neck Surgery, 106*, 175–80.

Ingram, R. E. (1990). Self-focused attention in clinical disorders: review and a conceptual model. *Psychological Bulletin, 107*, 156–176.

Jacob, R. G. (1988). Panic disorder and the vestibular system. *Psychiatric Clinics of North America, 11*, 361–374.

Jacob, R. G., Furman, J. M. R., Clark, D. B. and Durrant, J. D. (1992). Vestibular symptoms, panic and phobia: overlap and possible relationships. *Annals of Clinical Psychiatry*, 4, 163–174.

Jacob, R. G., Lilienfeld, S. O., Furman, J. M. R., Durrant, J. D. and Turner, S. M. (1989). Panic disorder with vestibular dysfunction: further clinical observations and description of space and motion phobic stimuli. *Journal of Anxiety Disorders, 3*, 117–130.

Jacob, R. G., Woody, S. R., Clark, D. B., Lilienfeld, S. O., Hirsch, B. E., Kucera, G. D., Furman, J. M. and Durrant, J. D. (forthcoming). Discomfort with space and motion: a possible marker of vestibular dysfunction assessed by the Situational Characteristics Questionnaire. *Journal of Psychopathology and Behavioural Assessment*.

Jacobs, J. (1992). Understanding family factors that shape the impact of chronic illness. In T. J. Akamatsu, M. A. P. Stephens, S. E. Hobfoll and J. H. Crowther (eds) *Family Health Psychology*. Washington, DC: Hemisphere Publishing Corporation.

Jacobson, N. S. and Truax, P. (1991). Clinical significance: a statistical approach to defining meaningful change in psychotherapy research. *Journal of Consulting and Clinical Psychology, 59*, 12–19.

Jakes, S. (1987). Psychological aspects of disorders of hearing and balance. In D. Stephens (ed.) *Adult Audiology: Scott-Brown's Otolaryngology (5th edn)*. London: Butterworths.

Jeans, V. and Orrell, M. W. (1991). Behavioural treatment of space phobia: a case report. *Behavioural Psychotherapy, 19*, 285–288.

Jones, D. R. and Hartman, B. O. (1984). Biofeedback treatment of airsickness: a review. In *Motion Sickness: Mechanisms, Prediction, Prevention and Treatment*. Proceedings of the AGARD symposium, May 1984, Williamsburg, Va, Loughton, AGARD.

Jones, D. R., Levy, R. A., Gardner, L., Marsh, R. W. and Patterson, J. C. (1985). Self-control of psychophysiologic response to motion stress: using biofeedback to treat airsickness. *Aviation, Space and Environmental Medicine, 56*, 1152–1157.

Jongkees, L. B. W. (1975). Positional nystagmus of the central type with particular reference to its clinical differentiation from the benign paroxysmal type. In R. F. Naunton (ed.) *The Vestibular System*. New York: Academic Press.

Kahane, J. and Auerbach, C. (1973). Effect of prior body experience on adaptation to visual displacement. *Perception and Psychophysics, 35*, 279–285.

Katz, A. E. (1986). Vertigo. In A. E. Katz (ed.) *Manual of Otolaryngology – Head and Neck Therapeutics*. Philadelphia, PA: Lea & Febiger.

Kemmler, R. W. (1984). Psychological components in the development and prevention of air sickness. In *Motion Sickness: Mechanisms, Prediction, Prevention and Treatment*. Proceedings of the AGARD symposium, May 1984, Williamsburg, Va, Loughton, AGARD.

Kerr, B., Condon, S. M. and McDonald, L. A. (1985). Cognitive spatial processing and the regulation of posture. *Journal of Experimental Psychology: Human Perception and Performance, 11*, 617–622.

Keshner, E. and Allum, J. H. J. (1986). Plasticity in pitch sway stabilization: normal habituation and compensation for peripheral vestibular deficits. In W. Bles and T. Brandt (eds) *Disorders of Posture and Gait*. Amsterdam: Elsevier.

Kirmayer, L. J. (1992). The body's insistence on meaning: metaphor as presentation and representation in illness experience. *Medical Anthropology Quarterly*, 6, 323–345.

Kleinman, A. (1986). Concepts and a model for the comparison of medical systems as cultural systems. In C. Currer and M. Stacey (eds) *Concepts of Health, Illness and Disease*. Leamington Spa: Berg.

Klosko, J. S., Barlow, D. H., Tassinari, R. and Cerny, J. A. (1990). A comparison of alprazolam and behavior therapy in treatment of panic disorder. *Journal of Consulting and Clinical Therapy*, 58, 77–84.

Kramer, A. and Spinks, J. (1991). Central nervous system measures of capacity. In J. R. Jennings and M. G. H. Coles (eds) *Handbook of Cognitive Psychophysiology*. Chichester: Wiley.

Kroenke, K. (1992). Symptoms in medical patients: an untended field. *American Journal of Medicine*, 92 (Suppl. 1A), 1A/35–1A/65.

Lawther, A. and Griffin, M. J. (1988). A survey of the occurrence of motion sickness amongst passengers at sea. *Aviation, Space and Environmental Medicine*, 59, 399–406.

Lazarus, R. S. (1991). *Emotion and Adaptation*. Oxford: Oxford University Press.

Lazarus, R. S., DeLongis, A., Folkman, S. and Gruen, R. (1985). Stress and adaptational outcomes: the problem of confounded measures. *American Psychologist*, 40, 770–779.

Leduc, A. and Decloedt, V. (1989). La kinesitherapie en O. R. L. *Acta Otorhinolaryngologica Belgica*, 43, 381–390.

Lee, W. A. (1989). A control systems framework for understanding normal and abnormal posture. *American Journal of Occupational Therapy*, 43, 291–301.

Leventhal, H., Meyer, D. and Nerenz, D. (1980). The common sense representation of illness danger. In S. Rachman (ed.) *Medical Psychology, Vol. 2*. New York: Pergamon.

Leventhal, H. and Mosbach, P. A. (1983). The perceptual-motor theory of emotion. In J. T. Cacioppo and R. E. Petty (eds) *Social Psychophysiology*. New York: Guilford Press.

Leventhal, H. and Nerenz, D. R. (1985). The assessment of illness cognition. In P. Karoly (ed.) *Measurement Strategies in Health Psychology*. New York: Wiley.

Levinson, H. N. (1989). A cerebellar-vestibular explanation for fears/phobias: hypothesis and study. *Perceptual and Motor Skills*, 68, 66–84.

Levy, I. and O'Leary, J. L. (1947). Incidence of vertigo in neurologic conditions. *Transactions of the America–Otologic Society*, 35, 329–347.

Ley, P. (1988). *Communicating with Patients*. London: Croom Helm.

Lilienfeld, S., Jacob, R. and Furman, J. (1989). Vestibular dysfunction followed by panic disorder with agoraphobia: a case report. *Journal of Nervous and Mental Disease*, 177, 700–702.

Linstrom, C. J. (1992). Office management of the dizzy patient. *Otolaryngologic Clinics of North America*, 25, 745–780.

Locker, D. (1981). *Symptoms and Illness: the Cognitive Organization of Disorder*. London: Tavistock.

Ludman, H. (1984). Surgical treatment of vertigo. In M. R. Dix and J. D. Hood (eds) *Vertigo*. Chichester: Wiley.

Luxon, L. M. (1984). Vertigo in old age. In M. R. Dix and J. D. Hood (eds) *Vertigo*. Chichester: Wiley.

Marks, I. M. (1981). Space 'phobia': a pseudo-agoraphobic syndrome. *Journal of Neurology, Neurosurgery and Psychiatry, 44*, 387–391.

Marks, I. M. (1987). *Fears, Phobias and Rituals*. Oxford: Oxford University Press.

Mauss, M. (1979). *Sociology and Psychology Essays*. London: Routledge & Kegan Paul.

McCabe, B. F. (1960). Vestibular suppression in figure skaters. *Transactions of the American Academy of Ophthalmology and Otology, 64*, 264–268.

McKenna, L., Hallam, R. S. and Hinchcliffe, R. (1991). The prevalence of psychological disturbance in neuro-otology outpatients. *Clinical Otolaryngology, 16*, 452–456.

McNally, R. J. (1990). Psychological approaches to panic disorder: a review. *Psychological Bulletin, 108*, 403–419.

Miller, S. M. (1979). Controllability and human stress: method, evidence and theory. *Behavioural Research and Therapy, 17*, 287–304.

Miller, S. M. (1990). To see or not to see: cognitive informational styles in the coping process. In M. Rosenbaum (ed.) *Learned Resourcefulness*. New York: Springer.

Mineka, S. and Kelly, K. A. (1989). The relationship between anxiety, lack of control and loss of control. In A. Steptoe and A. Appels (eds) *Stress, Personal Control and Health*. Chichester: Wiley.

Möller, C., Ödkvist, L., White, V. and Cyr, D. (1990). The plasticity of compensatory eye movements in rotatory tests I: The effect of alertness and eye closure. *Acta Otolaryngologica, 109*, 15–24.

Money, K. E. (1990). Motion sickness and evolution. In G. H. Crampton (ed.) *Motion and Space Sickness*. Boca Raton, Fla: CRC Press.

Morrison, A. W. (1984). Ménière's disease. In M. R. Dix and J. D. Hood (eds) *Vertigo*. Chichester: Wiley.

Morrow, G. R., Lindke, J.-L. and Black, P. M. (1991). Anticipatory nausea development in cancer patients: replication and extension of a learning model. *British Journal of Psychology, 82*, 61–72.

Nashner, L. M., Black, F. O. and Wall, C. (1982). Adaptation to altered support and visual conditions during stance: patients with vestibular deficits. *Journal of Neuroscience, 2*, 536–544.

Nashner, L. M., Shupert, C. L. and Horak, F. B. (1988). Head–trunk movement coordination in the standing posture. In O. Pompeiano and J. H. J. Allum (eds) *Vestibulospinal Control of Posture and Locomotion: Progress in Brain Research, Vol. 76*. Amsterdam: Elsevier.

Newman, F. L. and Howard, K. I. (1991). Introduction to the special section on seeking new clinical research methods. *Journal of Consulting and Clinical Psychology, 59*, 8–11.

Nicholas, M. K., Wilson, P. H. and Goyen, J. (1991). Operant-behavioural and cognitive-behavioural treatment for chronic low back pain. *Behaviour Research and Therapy, 29*, 225–238.

Nobbs, M. B. (1988). Adjustment in Ménière's disease. In J. G. Kyle (ed.) *Adjustment to Acquired Hearing Loss: Analysis, Change and Learning*, Proceedings of a conference held in University of Bristol, 9–13 April 1987. Bristol: Centre for Deaf Studies.

Norré, M. E. (1984). Treatment of unilateral vestibular hypofunction. In W. J. Oosterveld (ed.) *Otoneurology*. Chichester: Wiley.

Norré, M. E. (1988). Vestibular habituation training: specificity of adequate exercise. *Archives of Otolaryngology – Head and Neck Surgery, 114*, 883–886.

Norré, M. E. and Beckers, A. (1987). Exercise treatment for two types of paroxysmal positional vertigo: comparison of two types of exercises. *Archives of Otorhinolaryngology, 244*, 291–294.

Norré, M. E. and de Weerdt, W. (1980). Treatment of vertigo based on habituation. 2. Technique and results of habituation training. *The Journal of Laryngology and Otology, 94*, 971–977.

Norré, M. E., Forrez, G. and Stevens, M. (1984). Posturography and vestibular compensation. *Acta Otorhinolaryngologica Belgica, 38*, 619–631.

O'Connor, K. P., Chambers, C. and Hinchcliffe, R. (1989). Dizziness and perceptual style. *Psychotherapy and Psychosomatics, 51*, 169–174.

O'Connor, K. P., Hallam, R., Beyts, J. and Hinchcliffe, R. (1988). Dizziness: behavioural, subjective and organic aspects. *Journal of Psychosomatic Research, 32*, 291–302.

Ödkvist, I. and Ödkvist, L. M. (1988). Physiotherapy in vertigo. *Acta Otolaryngologica, 455 (Suppl.)*, 74–76.

Öhman, A. and Soares, J. J. F. (1993). On the automatic nature of phobic fear: conditioned electrodermal responses to marked fear-relevant stimuli. *Journal of Abnormal Psychology, 102*, 121–132.

Oosterveld, W. J. (1979). Ménière's disease, a survey of 408 patients. *Acta Otorhinolaryngologica Belgica, 33*, 428–431.

Oosterveld, W. J. (1984). Cervical vertigo. In W. J. Oosterveld (ed.) *Otoneurology*. Chichester: Wiley.

Osterhammel, P., Terkildsen, K. and Zilstorff, K. (1968). Vestibular habituation in ballet dancers. *Acta Otolaryngologica, 66*, 221–228.

Overstall, P. W. (1983). Rehabilitation of elderly patients with disorders of balance. In R. Hinchcliffe (ed.) *Hearing and Balance in the Elderly*. Edinburgh: Churchill Livingstone.

Page, N. G. R. and Gresty, M. A. (1985). Motorist's vestibular disorientation syndrome. *Journal of Neurology, Neurosurgery and Psychiatry, 48*, 729–735.

Paparella, M. M. (1991). Methods of diagnosis and treatment of Ménière's disease. *Acta Otolaryngologica, 485 (Suppl.)*, 108–119.

Paparella, M. M., Alleva, M. and Bequer, N. G. (1990). Dizziness. *Disorders of the Ears, Nose and Throat, 17*, 299–308.

Parnes, L. S. (1993). Benign paroxysmal positional vertigo: diagnosis and treatment. In J. A. Sharpe and H. O. Barber (eds) *The Vestibulo-ocular Reflex and Vertigo*. New York: Raven Press.

Pauli, P., Marquardt, C., Hartl, L., Nutzinger, D. O., Hotzl, R. and Strian, F. (1991). Anxiety induced by cardiac perceptions in patients with panic attacks: a field study. *Behaviour Research and Therapy, 29*, 137–145.

Pearce, S. and Erskine, A. (1989). Chronic pain. In S. Pearce and J. Wardle (eds) *The Practice of Behavioural Medicine*. Oxford: B.P.S. Books/Oxford University Press.

Pfaltz, C. R. (1984). Vertigo in disorders of the neck. In M. R. Dix and J. D. Hood (eds) *Vertigo*. Chichester: Wiley.

Pohl, D. V. (1991). Vestibular neurectomy: a review. *Journal of the Otolaryngological Society of Australia, 6*, 419–421.

Pollock, K. (1993). Attitude of mind as a means of resisting illness. In A. Radley (ed.) *Worlds of Illness*. London: Routledge.

Powers, W. T. (1973). *Behavior: the Control of Perception*. London: Wildwood House.

Pratt, R. T. C. and McKenzie, W. (1958). Anxiety states following vestibular disorders. *The Lancet, 2*, 347–349.

Pykkö, I., Magnusson, M., Schalén, L. and Enbom, H. (1988). Pharmacological treatment of vertigo. *Acta Otolaryngologica, 455 (Suppl.)*, 77–81.

Pyszczynski, T., Greenberg, J., Solomon, S. and Hamilton, J. (1991). A terror management analysis of self-awareness and anxiety: the hierarchy of terror. In R. Schwarzer and R. A. Wicklund (eds) *Anxiety and Self-focused Attention*. London: Harwood Academic Publishing.

Radley, A. (1993). The role of metaphor in adjustment to chronic illness. In A. Radley (ed.) *Worlds of Illness*. London: Routledge.

Rahe, R. H. (1988). Recent life changes and coronary heart disease: 10 years' research. In S. Fisher and J. Reason (eds) *Handbook of Life Stress, Cognition and Health*. Chichester: Wiley.

Raivio, M., Bunne, M. and Jorgensen, B. (1989). Evaluation of a three-stage management programme for Ménière's disease. *The American Journal of Otology, 10*, 443–446.

Rauch, S. D., Merchant, S. N. and Thedinger, B. A. (1989). Ménière's syndrome and endolymphatic hydrops: a double-blind temporal bone study. *Annals of Otology, Rhinology and Laryngology, 98*, 873–883.

RCGP/OPCS: Royal College of General Practitioners and Office of Population Census and Surveys (1986). *Morbidity Statistics from General Practice*. London: HMSO.

Reason, J. T. and Brand, J. J. (1975). *Motion Sickness*. New York: Academic Press.

Rigatelli, M., Casolari, L., Bergamini, G. and Guidetti, G. (1984). Psychosomatic study of 60 patients with vertigo. *Psychotherapy and Psychosomatics, 41*, 91–99.

Roberts, H. (1985). *The Patient Patients*. London: Pandora Press.

Robinson, I. (1988). *Multiple Sclerosis*. London: Routledge.

Rubinstein, B. and Erlandsson, S. I. (1991). A stomatognathic analysis of patients with disabling tinnitus and craniomandibular disorders (CMD). *British Journal of Audiology, 25*, 77–84.

Ruckenstein, M. J., Rutka, J. A. and Hawke, M. (1991). The treatment of Ménière's disease: Torok revisited. *Laryngoscope, 101*, 211–218.

Savundra, P., Breckenberg, J., Sutherland, R., Carter, J., Coelho, A., Davies, R. A., Mossman, S. and Luxon, L. M. (1993). A comparison of the Cawthorne–Cooksey exercises and relaxation therapy in the management of vertigo due to peripheral vestibular dysfunction. Paper presented at the 7th International Symposium on Audiological Medicine, Cardiff, 19–22 September.

Scambler, G. (1989). *Epilepsy*. London: Tavistock/Routledge.

Scheier, M. F. and Carver, C. S. (1988). A model of behavioral self-regulation:

translating intention into action. In L. Berkowitz (ed.) *Advances in Experimental Social Psychology, Vol. 21*. San Diego: Academic Press.

Schmidt, J. Th., and Huizing, E. H. (1992). The clinical drug trial in Ménière's disease with emphasis on the effect of betahistine SR. *Acta Otolaryngologica, 497 (Suppl.)*.

Schuknecht, H. F. (1975). Positional nystagmus of the benign paroxysmal type. In R. F. Naunton (ed.) *The Vestibular System*. New York: Academic Press.

Schwartz, G. E. (1982). Testing the biopsychosocial model: the ultimate challenge facing behavioral medicine? *Journal of Consulting and Clinical Psychology, 50*, 1040–1053.

Schwartz, G. E., Davidson, R. J. and Coleman, D. J. (1978). Patterning of cognitive and somatic processes in the self-regulation of anxiety: effects of mediation versus exercise. *Psychosomatic Medicine, 40*, 321–328.

Schwarzer, R. and Leppin, A. (1992). Possible impact of social ties on morbidity and mortality. In H. O. F. Veiel and V. Baumann (eds) *The Meaning and Measurement of Social Support*. New York: Hemisphere Publishing.

Schwarzer, R. and Wicklund, R. A. (eds) (1991). *Anxiety and Self-focused Attention*. London: Harwood Academic Publishers.

Selye, H. (1950). *Stress*. Montreal: Acta.

Shepard, N. T., Telian, S. A. and Smith-Wheelock, M. (1990). Habituation and balance training therapy. *Neurologic Clinics of North America, 8*, 459–475.

Shepard, N. T., Telian, S. A., Smith-Wheelock, M. and Raj, A. (1993). Vestibular and balance rehabilitation therapy. *Annals of Otology, Rhinology and Laryngology, 102*, 198–205.

Shumway-Cook, A. and Horak, F. B. (1989). Vestibular rehabilitation: an exercise approach to managing symptoms of vestibular dysfunction. *Seminars in Hearing, 10*, 96–108.

Skovronsky, O., Boleloucky, Z. and Baslecky, J. (1981). Anxiety and other neurotic symptoms in patients suffering from acoustic and vestibular disorders. *Agressologie, 22*, 25–26.

Smith, W. C. and Pillsbury, H. C. (1988). Surgical treatment of Ménière's disease since Thomsen. *The American Journal of Otology, 9*, 39–43.

Smyth, M. M., Pearson, N. A. and Pendleton, L. R. (1988). Movement and working memory: patterns and positions in space. *Quarterly Journal of Experimental Psychology, 41A*, 235–250.

Smyth, M. M. and Pendleton, L. R. (1989). Working memory for movements. *Quarterly Journal of Experimental Psychology, 40A*, 497–514.

Spitzer, J. B. (1990). An evaluation of the relationship among electronystagmographic, audiologic and self-report descriptors of dizziness. *European Archives of Otorhinolaryngology, 247*, 113–118.

Stacey, M. (1986). Concepts of health and illness and the division of labour in health care. In C. Currer and M. Stacey (eds) *Concepts of Health, Illness and Disease*. Leamington Spa: Berg.

Stahle, J., Friberg, U. and Svedberg, A. (1989). Long-term progression of Ménière's disease. *The American Journal of Otology, 10*, 170–173.

Stainton-Rogers, W. (1991). *Explaining Health and Illness*. New York: Harvester Wheatsheaf.

Stephens, S. D. G. (1975). Personality tests in Ménière's disorder. *Journal of Laryngology and Otology, 89*, 479–490.

Stephens, S. D. G. (1990). Auditory and vestibular rehabilitation in the adult. *Horizons in Medicine, 2*, 220–228.

Stephens, S. D. G., Hogan, S. and Meredith, R. (1991). The desynchrony between complaints and signs of vestibular disorders. *Acta Otolaryngologica, 111*, 188–192

Steptoe, A. and Appels, A. (eds) (1989). *Stress, Personal Control and Health*. Chichester: Wiley.

Stiles, W. B., Shapiro, D. A. and Elliott, R. (1986). 'Are all psychotherapies equivalent?' *American Psychologist, 41*, 165–180.

Stott, J. R. R. (1990). Adaptation to nauseogenic motion stimuli and its application in the treatment of airsickness. In G. H. Crampton (ed.) *Motion and Space Sickness*. Boca Raton, Fla: CRC Press.

Stott, J. R. R. and Bagshaw, M. (1984). The current status of the RAF programme of desensitisation for motion sick aircrew. In *Motion Sickness: Mechanisms, Prediction, Prevention and Treatment*, Proceedings of the AGARD symposium, May 1984, Williamsburg, VA. Loughton, England.

Takahashi, S., Fetter, M., Koenig, E. and Dichgans, J. (1990). The clinical significance of head-shaking nystagmus in the dizzy patient. *Acta Otolaryngologica, 109*, 8–14.

Taylor, S. E. (1983). Adjustment to threatening events: a theory of cognitive adaptation. *American Psychologist, 38*, 1161–1173.

Theunissen, E. J. J. M., Huygen, P. L. M. and Folgering, H. T. (1986). Vestibular hyperreactivity and hyperventilation. *Clinical Otolaryngology, 11*, 161–169.

Thompson, J. (1984). Communicating with patients. In R. Fitzpatrick, J. Hinton, S. Newman, G. Scambler and J. Thompson (eds) *The Experience of Illness*. London: Tavistock.

Thomsen, J., Bretlau, P., Tos, M. and Johnsen, N. J. (1983). Ménière's disease: a 3-year follow-up of patients in a double-blind placebo-controlled study on endolymphatic sac shunt surgery. *Advances in Oto-Rhino-Laryngology, 30*. Basel: Karger.

Toombs, S. K. (1992). *The Meaning of Illness*. Dordrecht: Kluwer.

Toscano, W. B. and Cowings, P. S. (1982). Reducing motion sickness: a comparison of autogenic feedback training and an alternative cognitive task. *Aviation, Space and Environmental Medicine, 53*, 449–453.

Triesman, M. (1977). Motion sickness: an evolutionary hypothesis. *Science, 197*, 493–495.

van den Berg, J. H. (1987). The human body and the significance of human movement. In J. J. Kockelmans (ed.) *Phenomenological Psychology: the Dutch School*. Dordrecht: Martinus Nijhoff.

Vasilyuk, F. (1991). *The Psychology of Experiencing*. London: Harvester Wheatsheaf.

Voorhees, R. L. (1989). The role of dynamic posturography in neurotologic diagnosis. *Laryngoscope, 99*, 995–1001.

Warwick, H. M. C. and Salkovskis, P. M. (1985). Reassurance. *British Medical Journal, 290*, 1028.

Watson, D. (1982). The actor and the observer: how are their perceptions of causality divergent? *Psychological Bulletin, 92*, 682–700.

Watson, D. and Pennebaker, J. W. (1989). Health complaints, stress and distress: exploring the central role of negative affectivity. *Psychological Review*, 96, 234–254.

Williams, J. M. G., Watts, F. N., Macleod, C. and Mathews, A. (1988). *Cognitive Psychology and Emotional Disorders*. Chichester: Wiley.

Woakes, E. (1896). *On Deafness, Giddiness and Noises in the Head* (4th edn). London: Lewis.

Wright, T. (1988). *Dizziness: a Guide to Disorders of Balance*. London: Croom Helm.

Yardley, L. (1991a). Orientation perception, motion sickness and vertigo: beyond the sensory conflict approach. *British Journal of Audiology*, 25, 405–413.

Yardley, L. (1991b). When your whole world is turned upside down: a mutualist analysis of vertigo and handicap. In P. J. Beek, R. J. Bootsma and P. C. W. Wieringen (eds) *Studies in Perception and Action*. Amsterdam: Rodopi.

Yardley, L. (1992). Motion sickness and perception: a reappraisal of the sensory conflict approach. *British Journal of Psychology*, 83, 449–471.

Yardley, L. (1994a). Contribution of symptoms and beliefs to handicap in people with vertigo: a longitudinal study. *British Journal of Clinical Psychology*, 33, 101–113.

Yardley, L. (1994b). Prediction of handicap and emotional distress in patients with recurrent vertigo: symptoms, coping strategies, control beliefs and reciprocal causation. *Social Science and Medicine* (in press).

Yardley, L. and Putman, J. (1992). Quantitative analysis of factors contributing to handicap and distress in vertiginous patients: a questionnaire study. *Clinical Otolaryngology*, 17, 231–236.

Yardley, L., Lerwill, H., Hall, M. and Gresty, M. (1992a). Visual destabilisation of posture. *Acta Otolaryngologica*, 112, 14–21.

Yardley, L., Masson, E., Verschuur, C., Luxon, L. and Haacke, N. P. (1992b). Symptoms, anxiety and handicap in dizzy patients: development of the Vertigo Symptom Scale. *Journal of Psychosomatic Research*, 36, 731–741.

Yardley, L., Todd, A. M., Lacoudraye-Harter, M. M. and Ingham, R. (1992c). Psychosocial consequences of vertigo. *Psychology and Health*, 6, 85–96.

Yardley, L., Verschuur, C., Masson, E., Luxon, L. and Haacke, N. P. (1992d). The influence of somatic and psychological factors on handicap and distress in patients with vertigo. *British Journal of Audiology*, 26, 283–291.

Yardley, L., Luxon, L. and Haacke, N. P. (1994a). A longitudinal study of symptoms, anxiety and subjective well-being in patients with vertigo. *Clinical Otolaryngology*, 19, 109–116.

Yardley, L., Luxon, L., Lear, S., Britton, J. and Bird, J. (1994b). Vestibular and posturographic test results in people with symptoms of panic and agoraphobia. *Journal of Audiological Medicine*, 3, 48–69.

Yardley, L., Gresty, M., Bronstein, A. and Beyts, J. (forthcoming). Changes in heart rate and respiration rate following head movements which provoke vertigo.

Zettle, R. D. and Hayes, S. C. (1982). Rule-governed behaviour: a potential theoretical framework for cognitive-behavioral therapy. In P. C. Kendall (ed.) *Advances in Cognitive-behavioral Research and Therapy, Vol. 1*. New York: Academic Press.

Name index

Subject index